first aid
in pictures

first aid in pictures

Dr. Robert Andrew

Illustrated by Ann Price-Owen

Wolfe

My grateful thanks to R. F. (Dick)
Herring, the best First Aid instructor
I know, for his help and co-operation
in the production of this book.

First published 1976 by
Wolfe Publishing Limited
10 Earlham Street
London WC2H 9LP

ISBN 0 7234 0463 1

Printed in Great Britain
by Ebenezer Baylis & Son Ltd
The Trinity Press, Worcester, and London

contents

duties of
first aid attendant

The duties of a first aid attendant are
solely to treat the conditions that he is
faced with, to prevent deterioration in
the general well-being of his patient,
relieve his anxiety and pain until such
time as medical help can be found. He
has two priorities
    1. To prevent the deterioration in
the general condition of the patient;
for example, by stopping the bleeding,
relieving pain and resuscitating.
    2. To seek expert medical aid, be
it a doctor, ambulance or transporting
to hospital, for the patient.
    These priorities must be kept in the
forefront of the first aider's mind all the
time. He should neither concentrate too
much on attending to the patient's injury
without seeking expert medical help, nor
should he neglect the patient and devote
all his energies to seeking expert help.
Depending on the condition or situation
he has to deal with, the priorities will
become clearer. There is always the
temptation to diagnose and treat, whereas
the role of the first aider is purely that of
holding the fort, doing the best he can
within the limits of his knowledge until
experts can take over with their skills
and facilities.

the scene of the accident

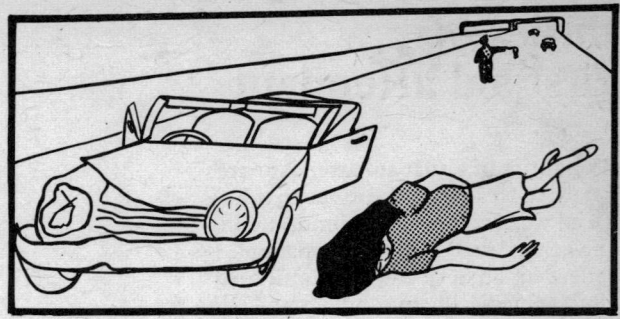

When arriving at the scene of an accident, the attendant's first duty is to make the accident situation secure: for example, it is no use rushing on to a motorway to attend a casualty if both of you are going to be run over; it is no good tying on a superb splint in a crumbling house if the house is going to fall both on you and your patient.

On arriving at the scene of an accident, assess the situation with the safety of the patient — from traffic, fire or falling debris being the main priorities. Not until then attend to the patient himself.

Typical situations that the attendant might have to deal with:
- *An injury on a roadway.* If the patient is not easily moveable, his first duty could be to go down the road and prevent traffic further endangering the situation.
- *A patient in an unsafe building.* Irrespective of his injuries it could be that the priority is to drag him clear before his injuries can be treated.
- *An unconscious patient in a gas-filled room.* The patient must be removed from the room, or the room cleared of gas before treatment can be commenced.

1   Attendant ensuring the safety of the accident situation.
2   Patient being removed from dangerous building, prior to treatment.
3   First aid attendant removing patient from gas-filled room.

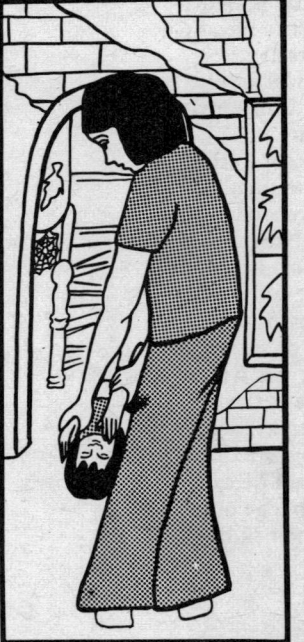

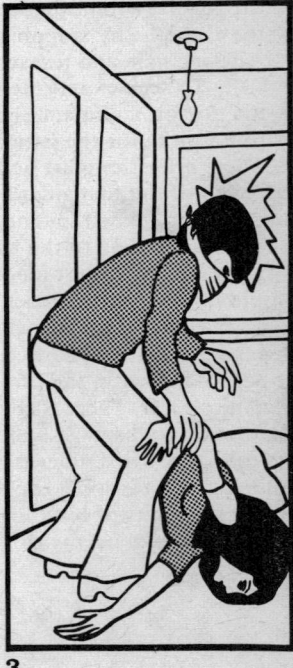

two minute first aid: general principles of major first aid treatment

bleeding

Control bleeding by applying direct pressure on bleeding area by either hand or a cloth pad. Press firmly to control bleeding. Where the bleeding is from a limb, assist the control of the bleeding by raising the limb as well as applying pad and pressure.

1 Applying pressure with pad on cut on wrist.
2 Raising the arm and applying pad where there has been a cut and bleeding.

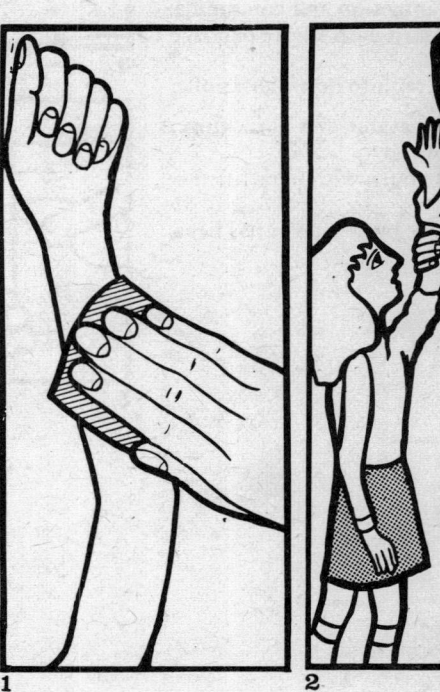

burns

The general principles for all burns are:
- Remove the patient from heat source.
- Take the heat out of the burn wherever possible by putting it under running water.
- Protect from infection and contamination, i.e. cover burn with sterile bandage or clean linen.

Severe burns require hospitalisation.

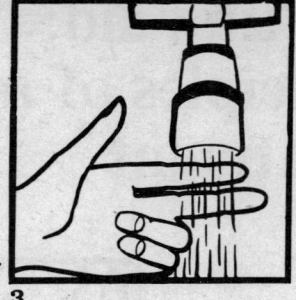
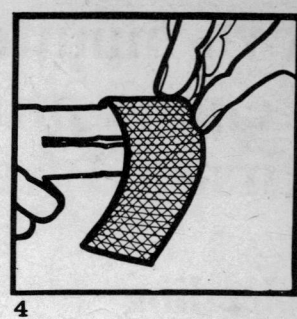

3   Taking the heat out of a burn, fingers under running water.
4   Covering the burn with paraffin gauze.
5   Bandaging the burn after it has been covered with the gauze.

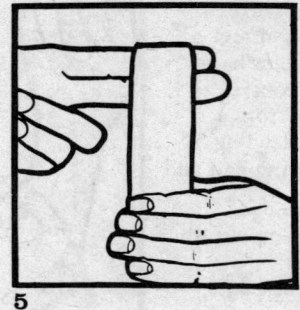

breaks and dislocations

Suspect a break or dislocation where there is pain and deformity of a limb or part of the body. Immobilise the limb, preventing the broken ends irritating or causing damage by tying the limb to a splint. In 80 per cent of all breaks the body can be used as a splint.

6   Deformity and pain in the right upper arm.
7 to 9   Immobilise the upper arm by splinting it to the body with series of pads and bandages.

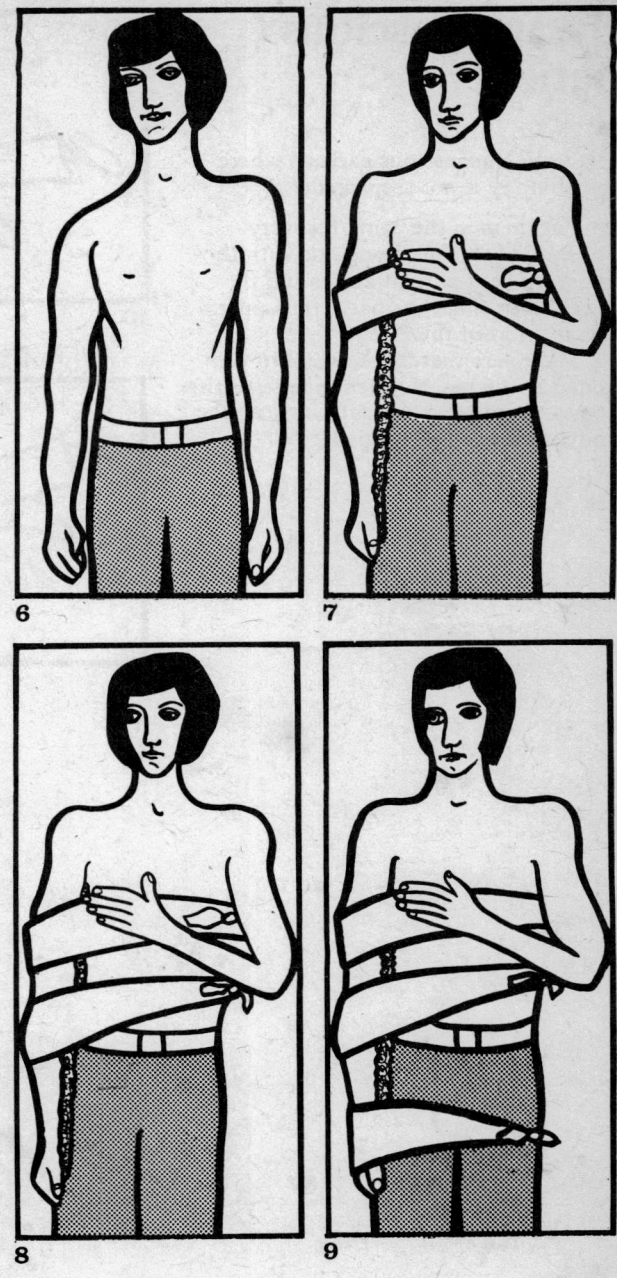

6 7 8 9

13

the unconscious patient

For all unconscious patients where spinal injury is not suspected:

10 Put them in the coma/recovery position, i.e. lying on one side with the upper leg bent at right angles and the lower arm behind the back, the upper arm in front of the face.

11 Make sure that there are no foreign bodies in the mouth, such as false teeth, vomit, mucus, etc. Air entering into the body must not be impeded.

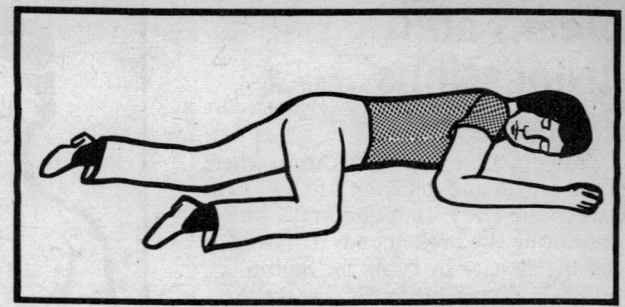

10

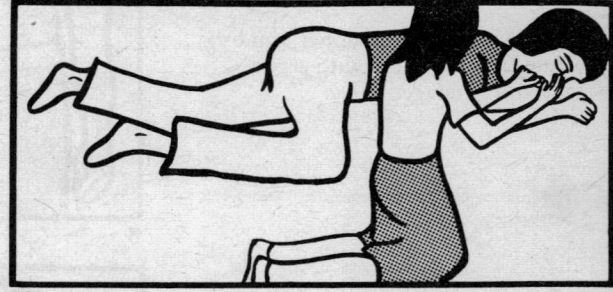

11

turning of casualty into the coma recovery position

This procedure disturbs the patient as little as possible.

12   Kneel beside the patient and place both his arms close to his body. Turn him gently on his side.

13   Draw up the upper arm until it makes a right angle to the body, and bend the elbow. Draw up the upper leg until the thigh makes a right angle to the body, and bend the knee.

14   Draw out the underneath arm gently backwards to bend down clear of the body.

15   Bend the undermost knee slightly. Make certain the head is kept on one side and the mouth is clear of mucus.

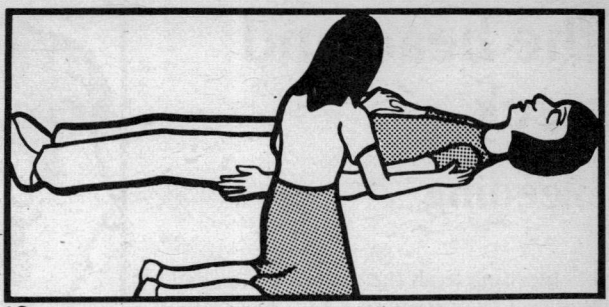

12

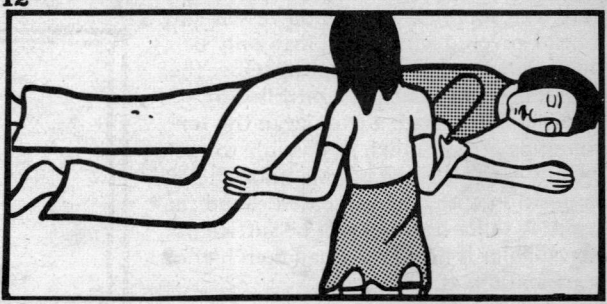

13

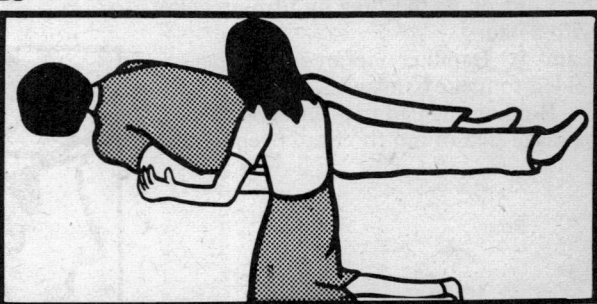

14

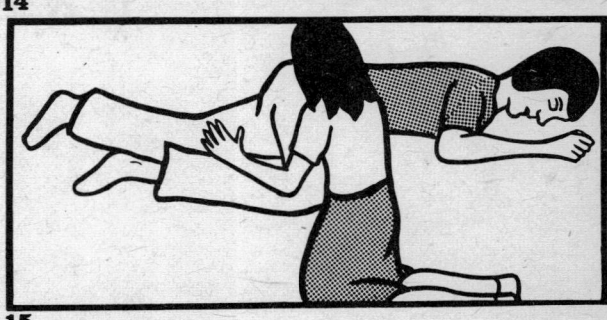

15

the head and neck

bleeding

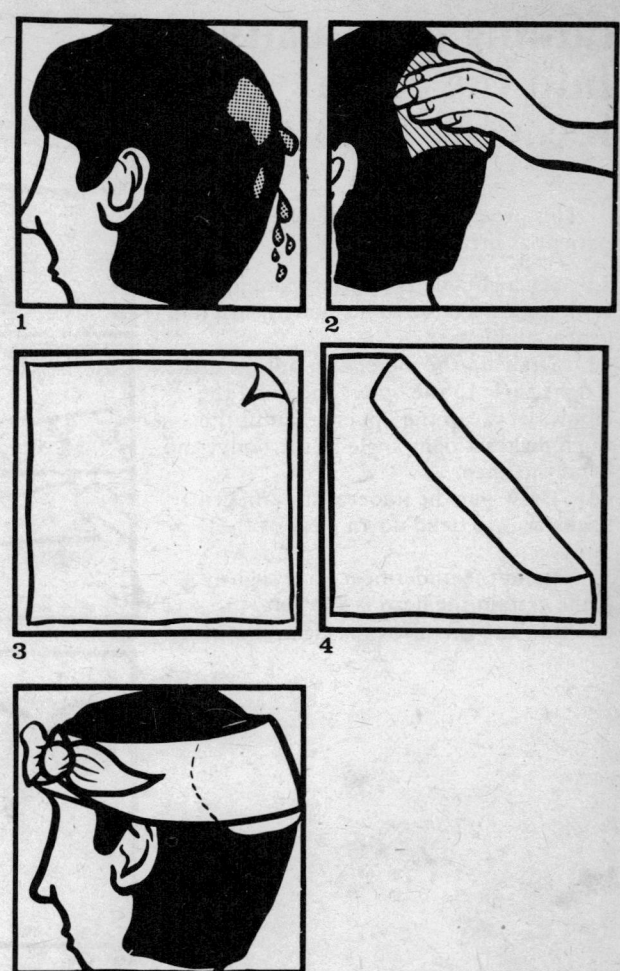

1   Bleeding from the scalp is controlled by direct pressure with a pad. The scalp is very well supplied with blood vessels and a head covered with blood may only be due to a minute cut on the scalp. Once the bleeding point has been controlled by pressing firmly with a pad, clean the surrounding area as much as possible to see exactly what is going on. Maintain the pad in position with a bandage tied round the scalp. A roller bandage will be sufficient if available: if not, fold a handkerchief or scarf and use as a bandage.

2   Controlling bleeding by firm pressure with a pad.
3 and 4   Handkerchief or scarf being folded to make bandage.
5   Holding the pad in position with a bandage tied round forehead over pad.

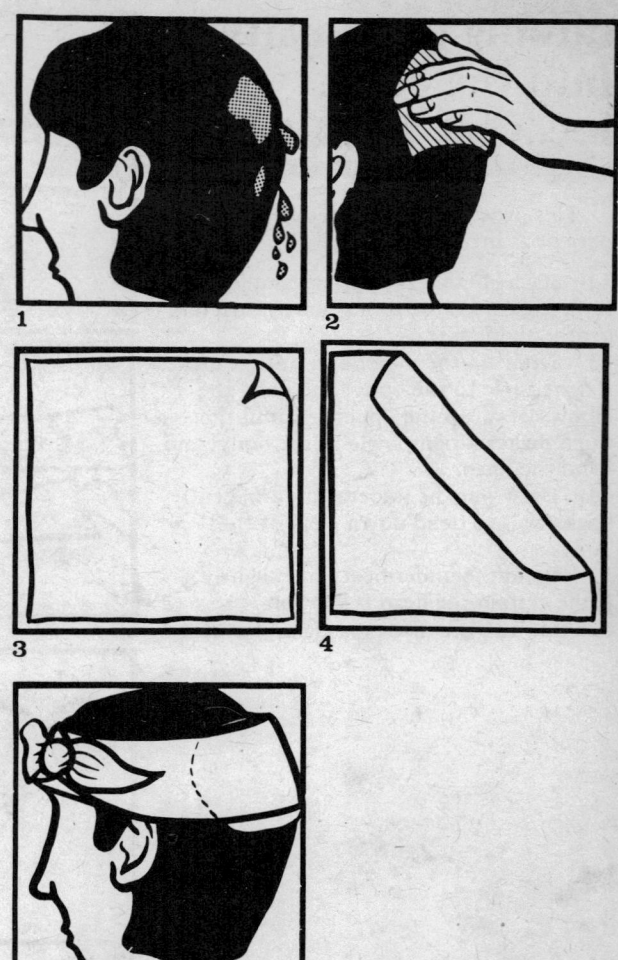

If a foreign body, such as a piece of glass, is stuck in the scalp and it cannot be removed easily, then a protective ring should be placed round the protruding object, then a pad applied overall and maintained in position with a bandage round the head.

6 to 9   To make the protective ring, fold a handkerchief or scarf from one corner to the other. Twist the folded handkerchief and twist the ends around each other.

The head bandage is best made by a triangular piece of material. This can be used either covering superficial head wounds or maintaining a ring pad in place.

10   Place a triangular bandage over the head, the broad base over the brow, the point at the back.
11   Bring the two ends to the back of the scalp.
12   Cross the two ends at the back and bring them and tie them on to the forehead.
13 and 14   Bring up tail of bandage and tie on top. The ring pad is under the head bandage.

continued overleaf

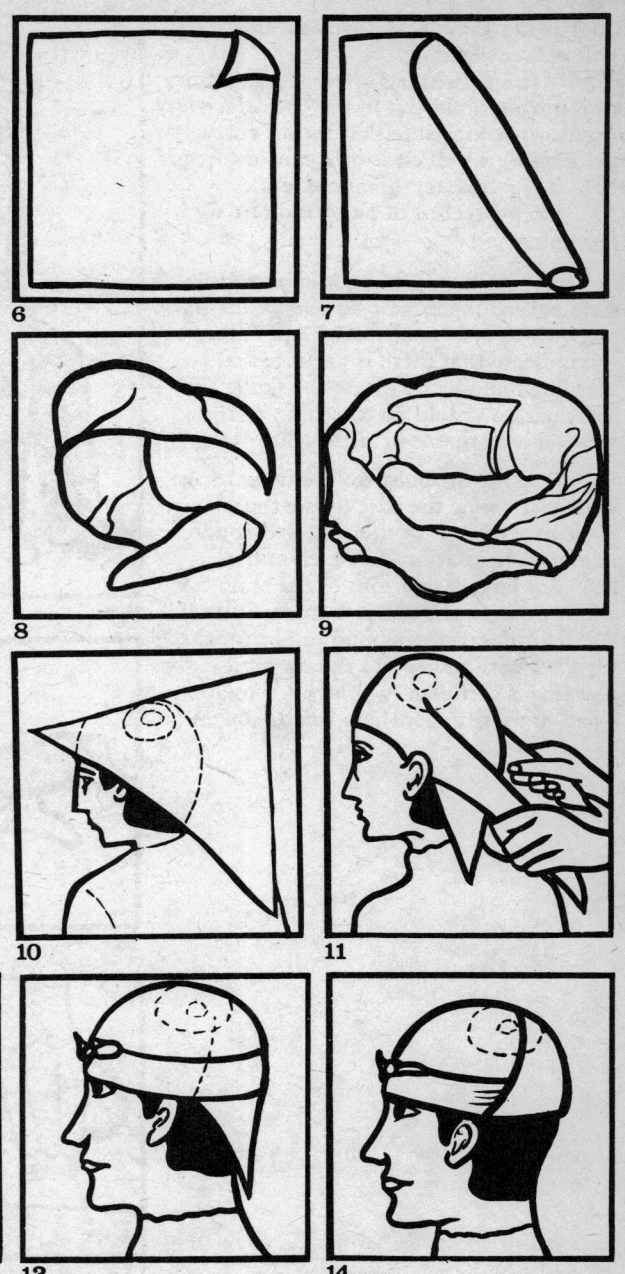

15 If the patient is conscious, sitting up will reduce bleeding.

16 If the patient has a severe head injury or is unconscious, put in the coma/recovery position, making sure that the air entry, i.e. mouth, is well clear of vomit or foreign bodies like false teeth, mucus, etc.

17 Keep a record of pulse and rate of breathing.

The recording of pulse is important in a serious head injury as a slowing of the pulse rate (which is normally 68–72 per minute) can indicate that there is pressure and bleeding building up inside the skull. This information should be passed on to the medical help that is being sought.

Feel for the pulse on the front of the wrist just below the base of the thumb. Place index finger in this area and count number of pulsations felt each minute.

18 For large lacerations of the scalp where a single pad will not control bleeding, the sides of the wound can be pinched together with finger and thumb until bleeding is sufficiently controlled to apply a pad or more expert help can be sought.

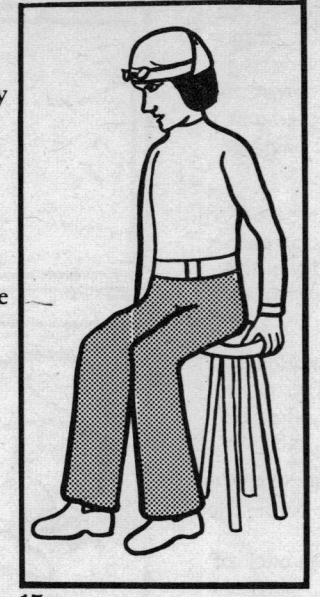

15

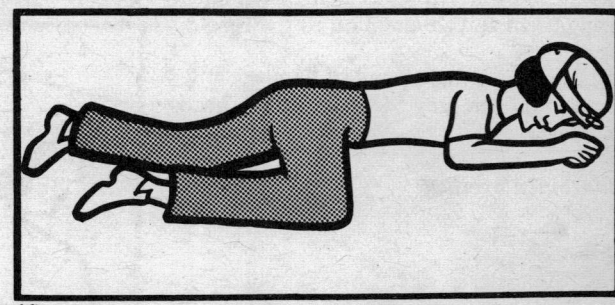

16

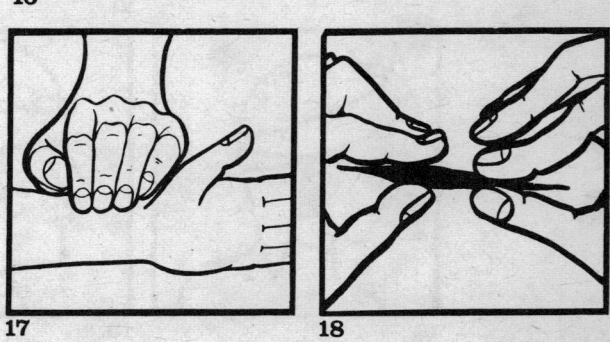

17   18

bleeding from the nose

1 and 2   Bleeding from the nose is rarely a sign of any serious medical condition. It is controlled by pinching the nose just below the bony structure with finger and thumb. Most often the patient can be instructed to do this himself. He should be leaning slightly forward, breathing through the mouth. The nose should be held for 10 minutes. If, on releasing pressure, there is a recurrence of bleeding, then the nose should be held for a further 20 minutes.

3 and 4   If the bleeding has still not stopped, the nose should be packed with a ribbon bandage or handkerchief strips, packing up both nostrils as high as one can, using ordinary tweezers and gripping the nose again after it has been packed.

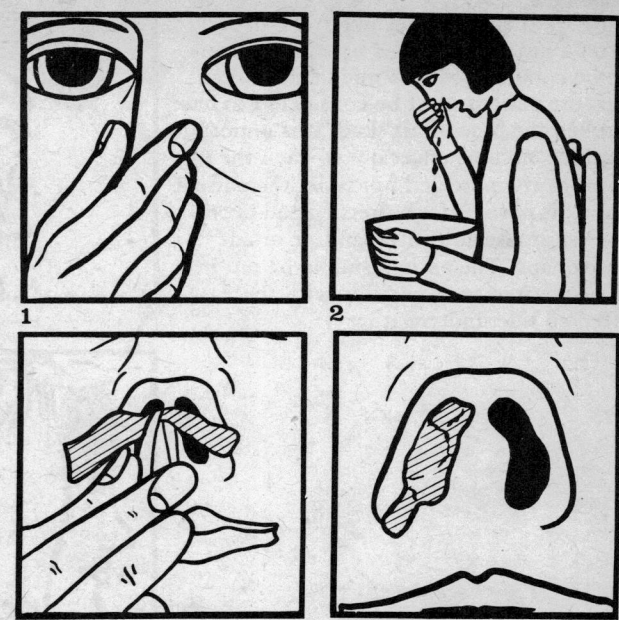

bleeding from the ear

1 to 3   For small surface cuts treat by applying a pressure pad and fixing the pad in place with a bandage round the scalp.

continued overleaf

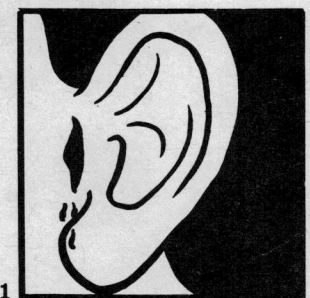
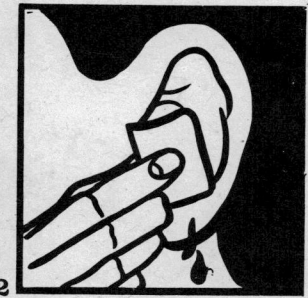
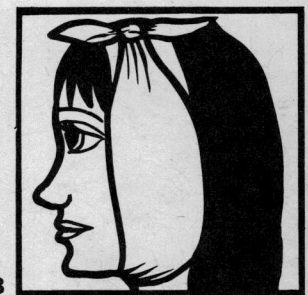

19

4 to 7   If there is bleeding from an ear
after a head injury, or if bleeding appears
to be coming from the middle part of an
ear, the patient must be considered to have
broken the base of his skull. It is important
in these circumstances not to pack the ear
canal or the nose and not to let the patient
blow his nose. Place a dressing pad over
the ear and secure with bandage or adhesive tape. The patient should be put in
the coma/recovery position with the
affected side underneath.

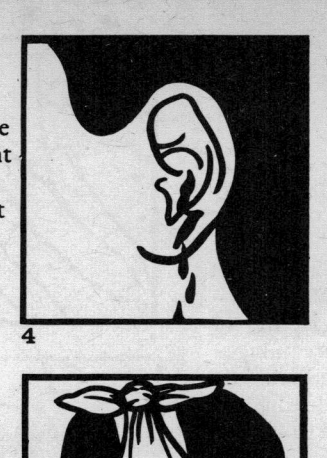

4

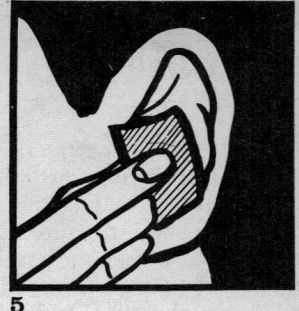

5

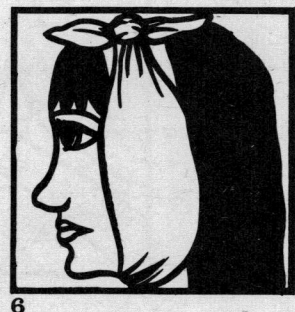

6

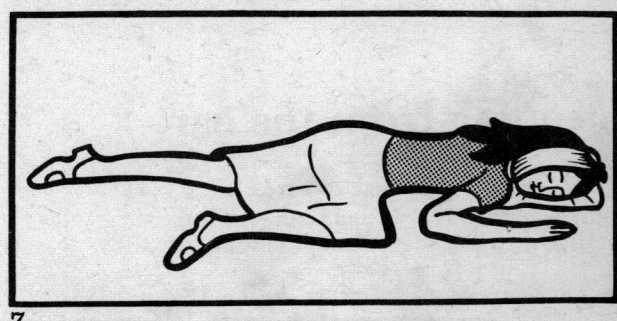

7

bleeding
from the mouth

1 to 3   Where the cause of bleeding from the mouth is obvious, such as following a dental extraction, a blow, or cut, and the patient can move his jaw properly and there is nothing to indicate that the jaw is broken, let the patient bite on a roll bandage, applying direct pressure to the bleeding area.

4 and 5   Where the teeth are damaged, check that all fragments of tooth are accounted for, in case during the blow that caused the teeth to be broken the patient has taken a piece of tooth into his lungs.

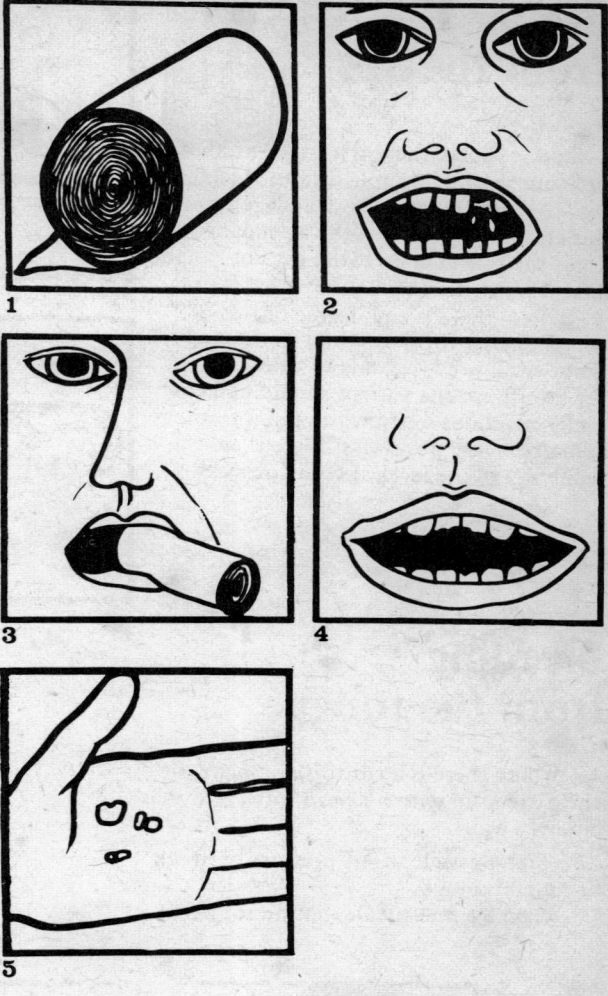

21

bleeding
from the lips

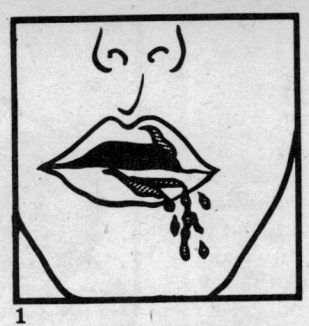
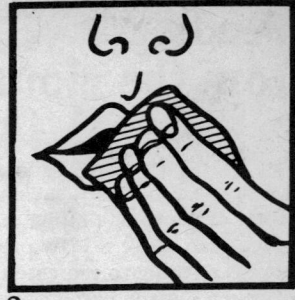

1 and 2   Where there is a large cut, direct pressure should be applied to the bleeding area. It is difficult to fix a bandage round this area and it is best if the attendant holds the pad in place if the patient cannot hold it himself.

3   Where there is any degree of loss of consciousness it is important that blood is not swallowed or going to the back of the mouth, so the patient should be kept under strict observation and put into the coma/recovery position if there is any reduction in the level of consciousness.

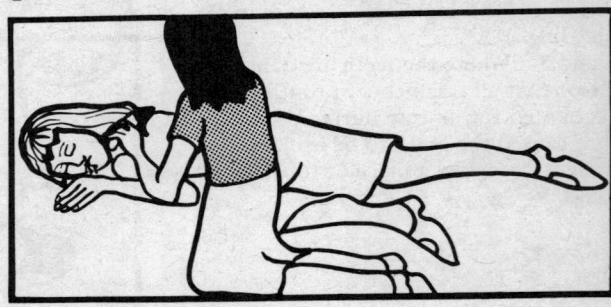

bleeding
from the tongue

1   Where there is a cut to the tongue, sit the patient up with his head forward over a bowl.

2   When possible, exert pressure between finger and thumb.

3   When ice is available, put on ice pack.

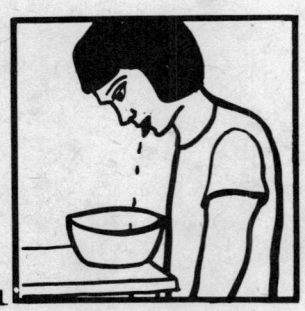
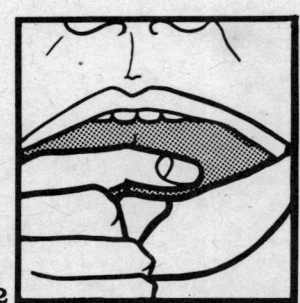
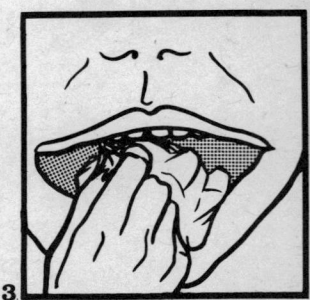

If there is no obvious injury, and still bleeding from the mouth, suspect that this could be:

● Blood dripping from the nose into the back of the throat.

● Blood from the lungs, where it would be coughed up and would be red and frothy and would be likely to be associated with some pain in the chest or cough.

● From the stomach, where it would be brown and like coffee-grounds. It would be vomited up, and there would be some history of vomiting and/or abdominal pain. One would have to act accordingly, depending on what conclusion one came to as to the source of the bleeding.

bleeding from the eyes

1 and 2   Any bleeding from the eyeball is an indication for rapid transfer of the patient to hospital. In the meantime protect the eye from contamination and infection by covering it with a dressing and bandage. The dressing should be loosely applied to the eye so as to exert no pressure on it.

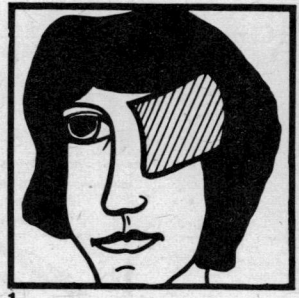 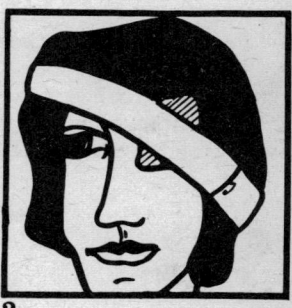

foreign bodies in the eye

1   For pieces of grit, flies, etc., that get into the eye, try and remove by washing out, that is to say, gently pouring water over the eyeballs, with the head on one side and the upper lid pulled up.

2   If the foreign body still remains, it may be gently probed with soft tissue such as a handkerchief. Great care should be taken not to scratch the eye and if there is any resistance, do not attempt to force the foreign body out.

3   A pad being applied to the eye.

4   A simplified bandage going once round the head, holding the pad over the eye.

5   For grit and foreign bodies under the eyelids, roll up the upper eyelid with a matchstick or orange stick.

6   Flush out with water; then roll the upper eyelid over the lower eyelid.

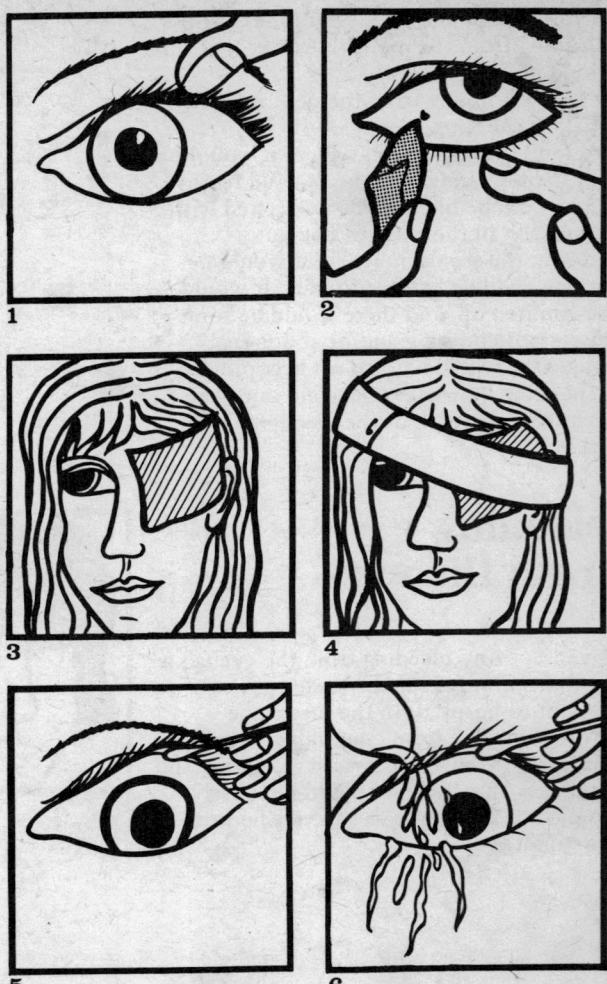

24

bleeding from the neck

1 and 2   Bleeding from any laceration to the the neck should be controlled by direct pressure with a pad. If, as in the case of attempted suicide, there is a large cut, one must be careful when applying pressure to apply the maximum pressure that does not interfere with other functions of the neck, such as breathing and swallowing. Having applied a bandage to the neck, keep it in position by tying round with a bandage as tightly as possible without constricting swallowing or breathing mechanisms.

3 and 4   Cuts to the neck are usually across the neck and severe bleeding is often best controlled by nipping the sides of the wound together with finger and thumb.

5   Where there is considerable loss of blood and possible unconsciousness, put the patient in the coma/recovery position, dress wound and observe.

When the patient is conscious and lucid, keep him in an upright position to help reduce the bleeding.

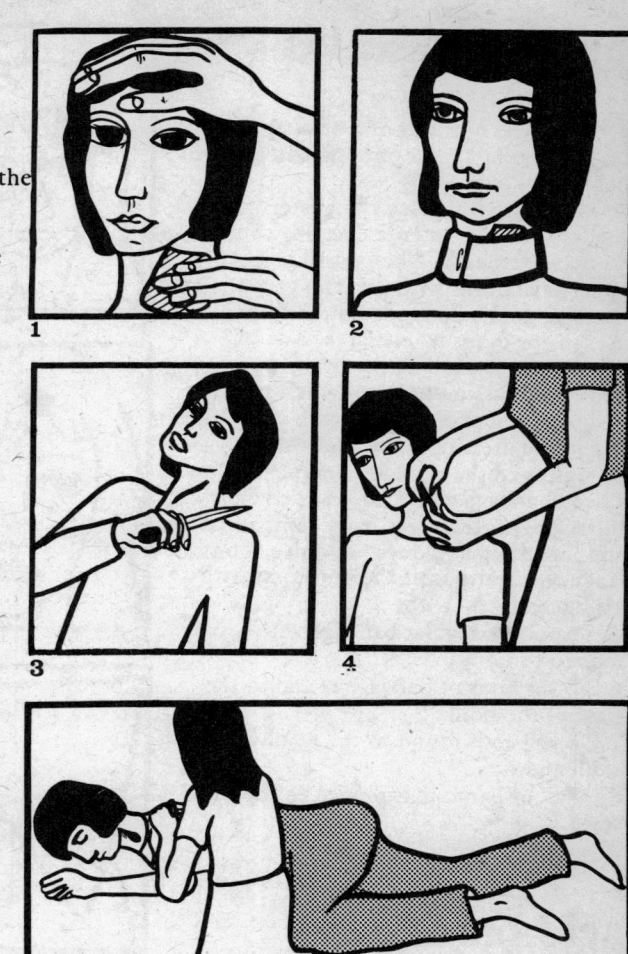

burns and scalds

1   Take the heat out of a burn by putting under running tap or pouring a stream of cold water over.

2 and 3   Do not prick the blisters. Blisters provide a sterile covering to the tissue underneath. When possible treat superficial burns with paraffin gauze dressing applied directly to the skin. For major burns where large areas of body tissue, including the head, are involved, admission to hospital is a priority, keeping the burns covered with clean linen if a sterile dressing is not available.

4   Burns to the head are best covered by a head bandage which covers the whole of the scalp, protecting it from contamination and infection, and does not move about. Take the heat out of the burn first with cold water.

5   Apply triangular bandage with broad side to forehead.

6   Bring ends of bandage round to the base of the skull.

7   Bring ends round to the front of the skull and tie.

8   Tail of bandage is pinned to top of scalp.

acid burns to the eyes

Acid burns to the eyes should be washed out immediately, i.e. cold water poured over them in volume, and covered, and patient rushed immediately to hospital.

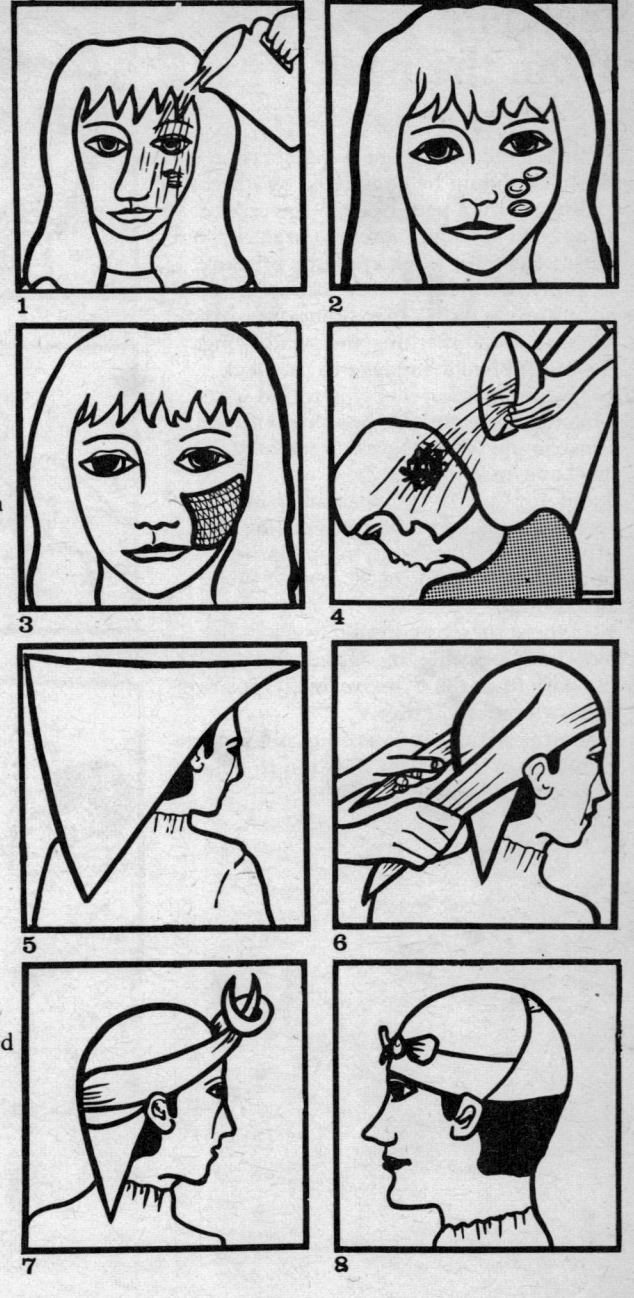

burns to the mouth

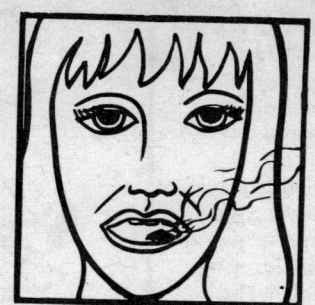

Inspect the mouth following the intake of hot liquids to ensure that the airway is not swollen or obstructed.

1   Corrosive burns of the mouth require immediate hospital attention. They are recognised by discolouration of the mouth, gums and tongue. Do not give fluids by mouth. Where possible identify the substance that has been swallowed to help with the hospital treatment of patient, and get the patient to hospital as quickly as possible.

breaking bones in the head and neck

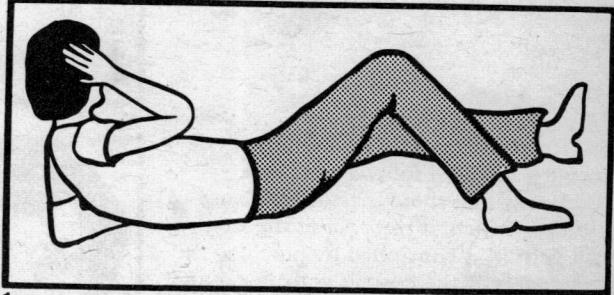

1   Do not attempt to decide whether the *skull* has been broken or not. If the head has suffered a severe blow, one has to prove not that the patient has a break in the bone, but to make certain that he has not. If at any time there is any doubt, only an x-ray of the skull can prove whether there is a break or not. In any head injury one should look out for the signs of bleeding inside the skull, the only signs of which may be progressive loss of consciousness, slowing of the pulse rate and possibly vomiting.

2   Patient with obvious injury to skull, bleeding from the ear, indicating a break in the base of the skull.

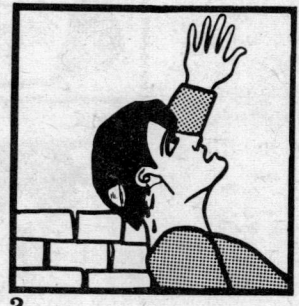

continued overleaf

3 In the circumstances where a break in the skull is suspected, if the patient is conscious put him in a comfortable position in a semi upright posture, keeping a close eye on pulse, respiration and level of consciousness.

4 If the patient does become unconscious he should be put into the coma/recovery position and if there is bleeding from one ear at the same time, put a loose dressing over the ear and put the patient in the coma/recovery position with the bleeding ear underneath.

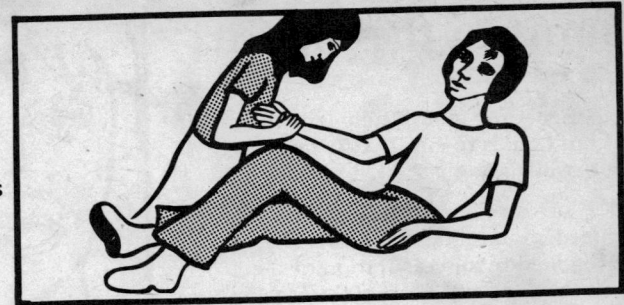

3

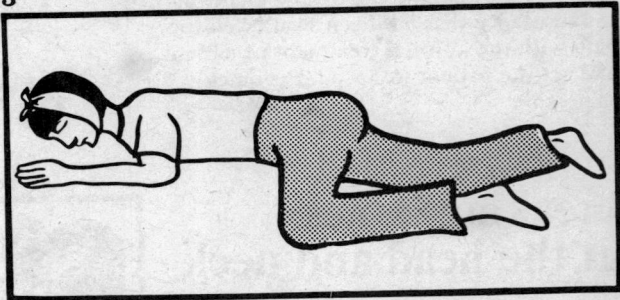

4

5 Recognise a *break in the nose* by deformity and pain following a blow.

6 Very often there is associated nose bleeding which, if the pain of the nose will permit, is controlled by pinching the lower ends of the nostrils with finger and thumb. Generally injuries to the nose do not cause serious complications, but the injured area should be protected and will require hospital examination by x-ray.

7 Patient with broken, bleeding nose, controlling bleeding by sitting up, head forward, breathing through the mouth, pinching nostril between finger and thumb.

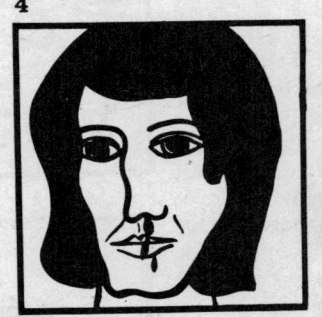

5

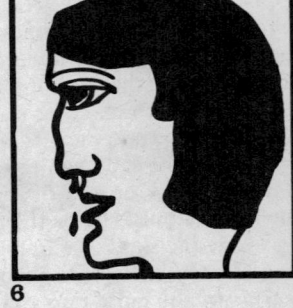

6

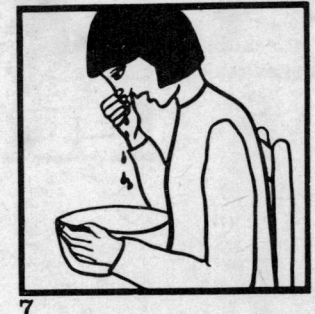

7

8   Injuries to the *bony structure round the eye*, with or without bleeding. Where there is a possibility of a break, it should be x-rayed. Pain and swelling in the area following a blow would make you suspect there had been bone injury.

9 and 10 If there is swelling round the eye, for the patient's comfort it is better to cover the eye with a pad and bandage.

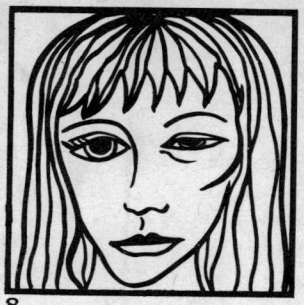

8

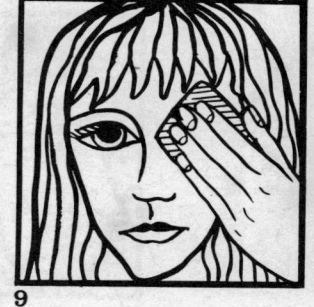

9

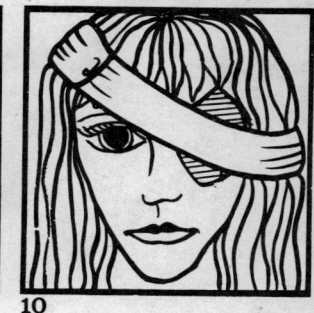

10

11   Pain and deformity of the jaw following injury suggests that the *jaw is broken*. Three points to look for: irregularity of the line of the teeth; downward displacement of the jaw; difficulty in the movement of the jaw.

12   Depending on the circumstances of the patient, the broken jaw is treated by splinting the jaw to the head. If the jaw is the only injury received by the patient, it is sometimes sufficient for him to hold it in the maximum position of comfort by fixing it with his hands.

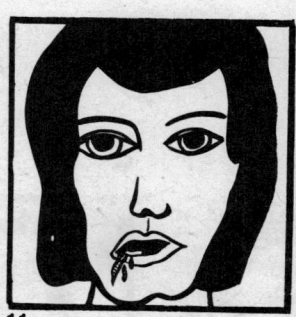

11

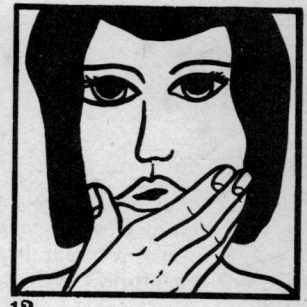

12

continued overleaf

13 The jaw can be fixed by placing a pad under the jaw and looping a bandage back over the top of the head.

14 Anchor it with a bandage at right angles round the brow.

15 Make the final tie on the temple. Great care must be taken if there is any bleeding from the mouth and one is fixing the jaw that the patient is not in any danger of inhaling blood.

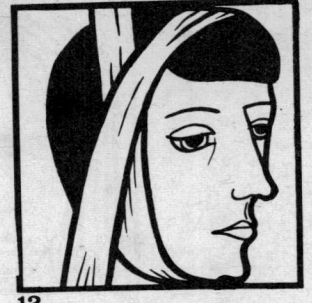

13

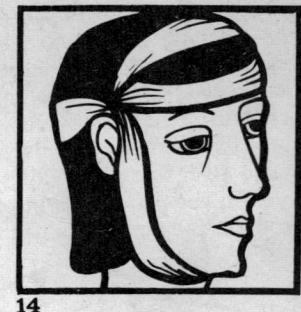

14

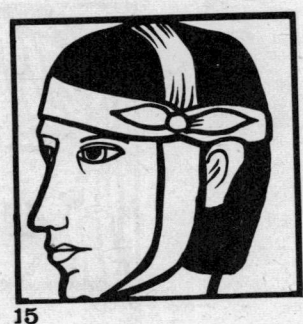

15

16 A *broken neck* must be suspected when there is an injury to the neck and the patient complains of paralysis or loss of power and sensation in the limbs. Similarly, if the patient is unconscious and the line of the neck is deformed, this suggests that there has been a break or dislocation of the spinal vertebrae of the neck. The first aider's duty is to move the patient as little as possible, undo restrictive clothing such as ties, neck buttons, support the neck with padding, cushions and blankets, so that there is no movement in any direction, i.e. support from all sides.

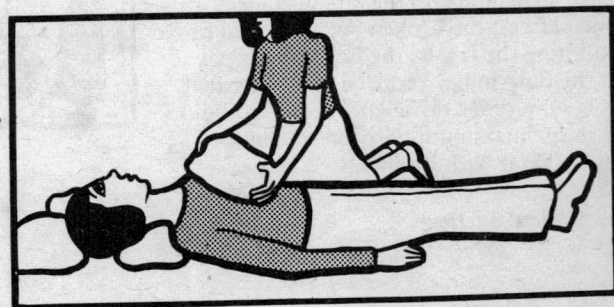

16

If the situation is such that the patient has to be removed from a dangerous situation before expert medical help can arrive, the patient should be moved completely supported in all positions so that there is no movement of one part of the body on another.

17　Patient with limbs tied together, head supported, being prepared to roll.

18　Patient rolled, with blanket folded underneath.

19　Patient on blanket being lifted on to stretcher.

The patient, once on the stretcher, should be transported to hospital as gently and smoothly as possible, with the neck padded so that there is no movement.

(See *Transport of Patient,* page 156)

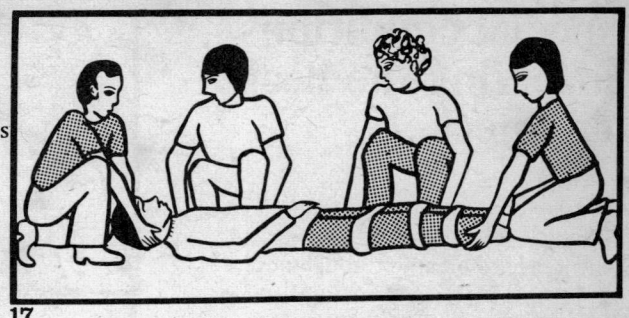

17

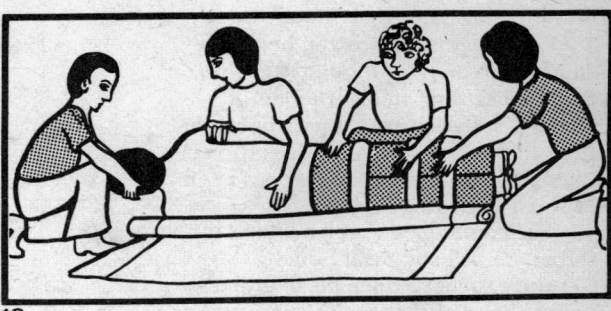

18

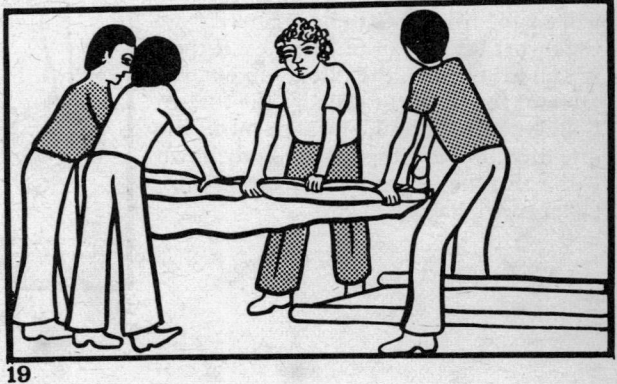

19

special conditions affecting the head and neck

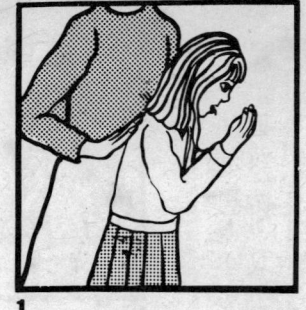

1   *Choking* with foreign body or food in the throat. Reassure the patient and encourage to breathe through nose.

2   If making no progress, hit in the back. For a child lay over the knee and hit on the back.

3   Put finger in mouth and hook out any foreign body or food matter that might be causing an obstruction. If choking not relieved, get patient on the floor on his side so that resuscitation or thumping the back will ensure safe exit of foreign choking material.

4   The commonest foreign bodies in the throat are fish and meat bones.
Get the patient to open his mouth, and inspect back of the throat, depressing the tongue with a spoon. Sometimes this will enable fish bones to be removed from the throat with a pair of tweezers. If there is pain lower down the throat, do not attempt to remove or dislodge the foreign body by eating bread, etc. Seek medical attention. Forcing the foreign body down with soft food may cause damage to the gullet (oesophagus).

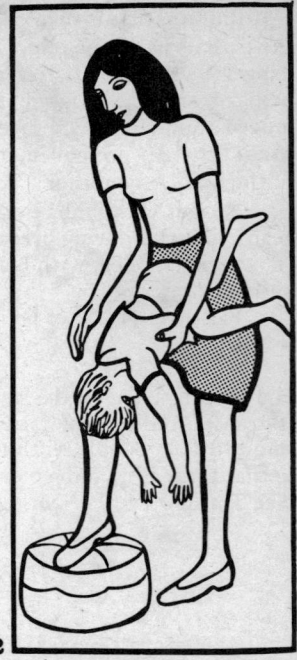

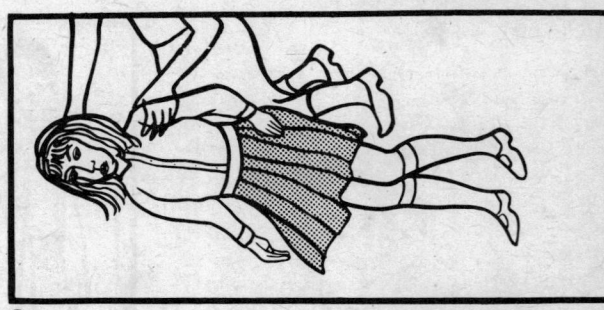

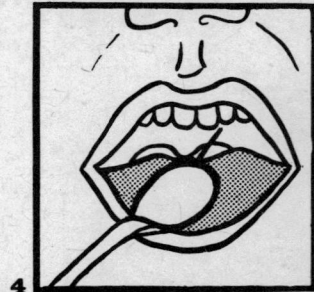

5 Foreign bodies in the *ear* occur particularly in children — they are usually beads or sweets or, in some cases, with children and adults, small insects can get in. Do not probe into ears to try and remove foreign bodies. If it cannot be floated out by tipping water into the ear, it must be removed by a doctor or nurse with a proper medical syringe.

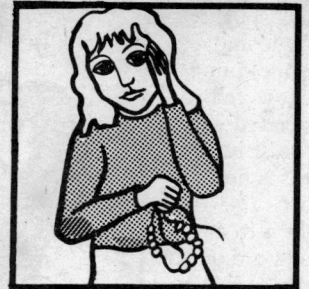

5

6 and 7 Following a blow to the head, where there has been loss of consciousness, however temporary, or if the patient does not in any way seem to be himself or has loss of memory, he should be treated as a case of *concussion*. The patient should be at complete rest until more expert medical opinion can be found, and the pulse and rate of breathing, level of consciousness watched closely. The general condition of the patient and his mental outlook should be noted, i.e. is he getting more drowsy and confused? Is he staying the same or is he getting better?

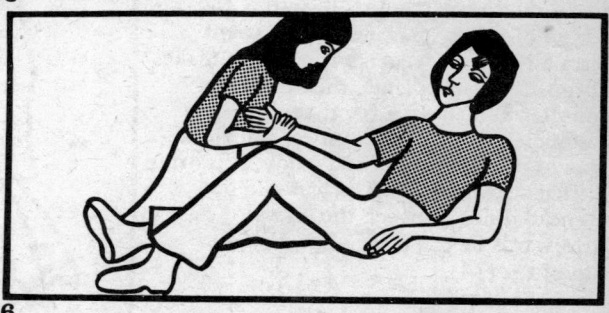

6

8 With *strokes and cerebral haemorrhage* there has been clotting of blood in a vessel in the brain or the bursting of a blood vessel in the brain. The onset is usually sudden; the patient may be conscious or unconscious; there will be paralysis, usually on one side. It must be remembered that if the patient has difficulty in speaking, it is also likely that half the swallowing muscles are paralysed and the patient should not be given drinks as they could go straight into the lungs, causing a failure in breathing.

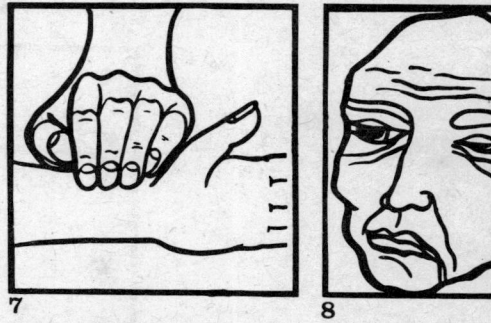

7

8

9 Treat as for the unconscious patient, that is to say, put in the coma/recovery position on his side, making sure that the breathing airway is not obstructed. Look for deterioration in the general condition of the patient by checking the pulse rate, the rate of breathing and the level of consciousness and co-operation.

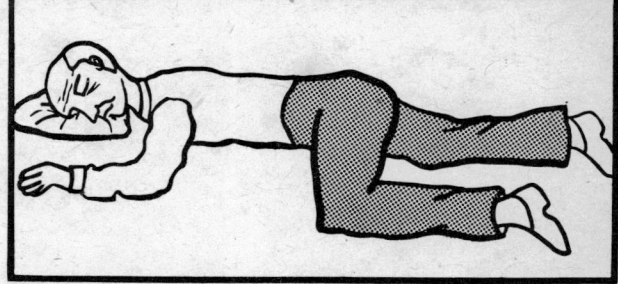

9

continued overleaf

10 to 14 *Fainting* can occur at all ages, the patient suddenly losing consciousness. They usually come round very quickly when the head is lowered. Most often fainting is not associated with any serious bodily illness but must be observed closely to see that this is not a fit. There is a temporary loss of consciousness when the patient is in an upright position. The patient should be put into the coma/recovery position (13) and should soon recover. If, during the period of unconsciousness, the patient bites his tongue, wets his trousers or makes purposeless movements, then one must consider that this is a fit. If there is no complete loss of consciousness and the patient just feels weak and giddy, it is often sufficient to sit him on a chair and put his head down between the knees. Afterwards he can have a hot, sweet cup of tea (14).

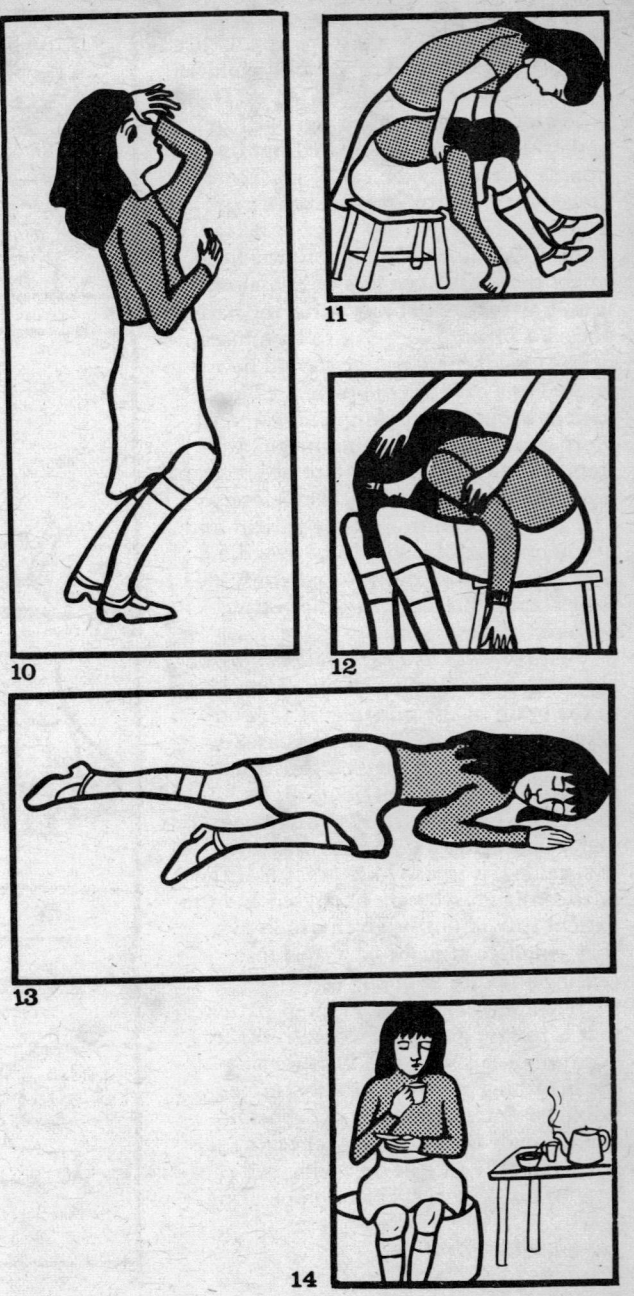

first aid treatment of the unconscious patient

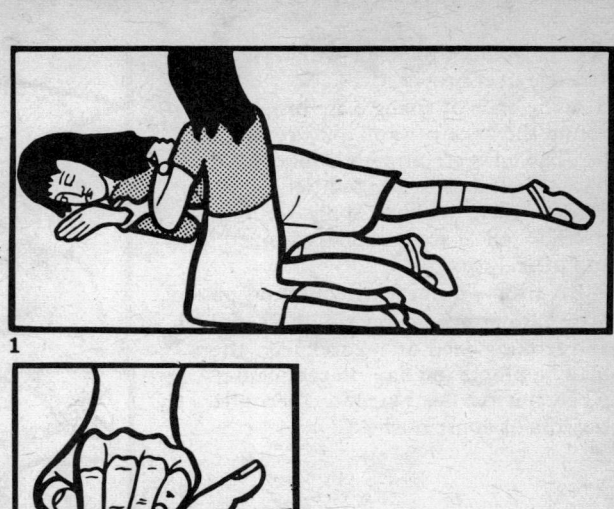

1   Remember that the unconscious patient is a serious medical emergency and expert medical help should be sought at the earliest possible opportunity. First assess the patient. Observe the rate of pulse, the strength of the pulse, the rate of breathing, and the colour of the patient, whether he is pink or blue, blueness of the lips being a sign that he is not breathing efficiently. Lay the patient in the coma/recovery position, examine the mouth to see that the airway is clear, and remove any false teeth, vomit or saliva.

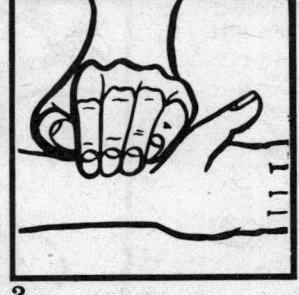

2   Assess the patient. Observe the rate of pulse, the strength of the pulse, the rate of breathing, and the colour of the patient, whether he is pink or blue, blueness of the lips being a sign that he is not breathing efficiently.

3   The first aider should then try and assess the cause of unconsciousness. In finding out, it is helpful to consider:

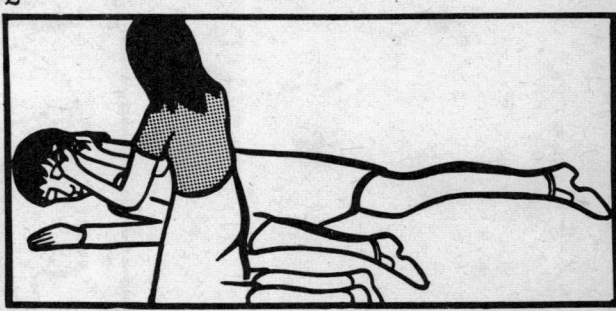

● Is there a head wound which would make a blow to the head the likely cause?
● At the same time consider that the head wound could be a secondary cause: if the patient has hit his head after falling there should be some evidence to suggest which of the two is the more likely.

Treat any injury such as scalp wounds for bleeding, etc.

continued overleaf

4 Apply head bandage with base of triangle over brow.

5 The ends of triangle are brought round the back of skull and crossed.

6 The ends are brought round from back of skull to brow, and tied.

7 The scalp bandage in position.

8 The tail of scalp bandage pinned on top of scalp.

9 A scalp wound to unconscious patient.

10 Patient losing consciousness, falling and striking head on mantelpiece, there may be blood and hair on the mantelpiece, but the head wound is secondary to the loss of consciousness.

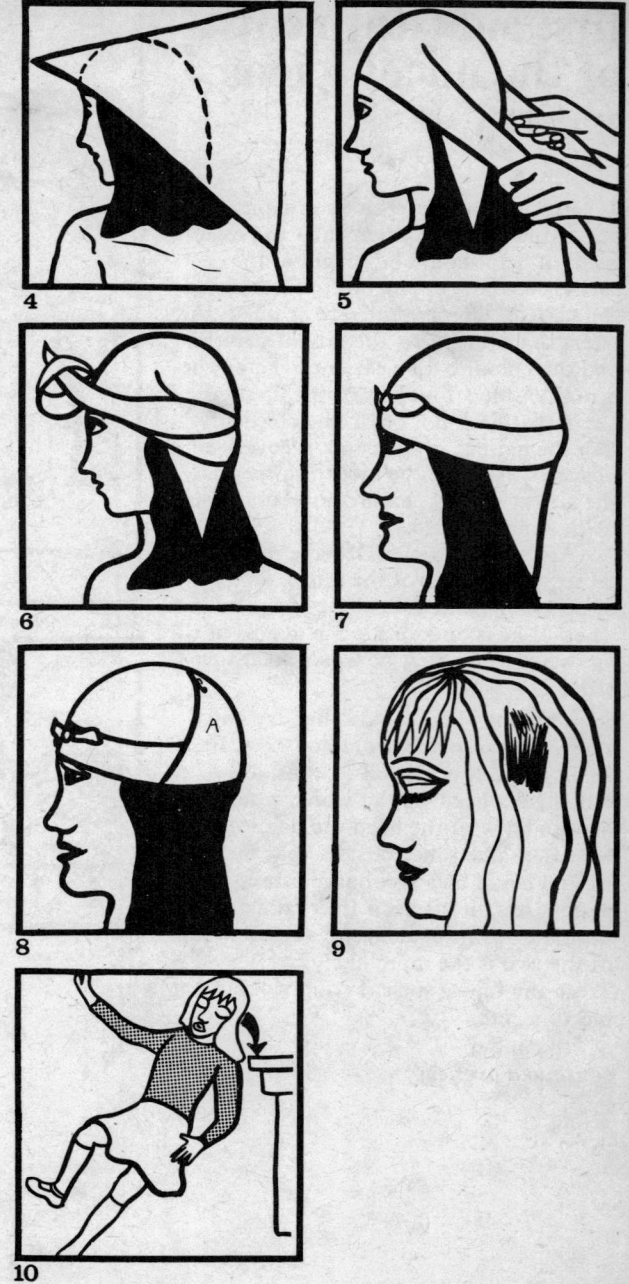

fits

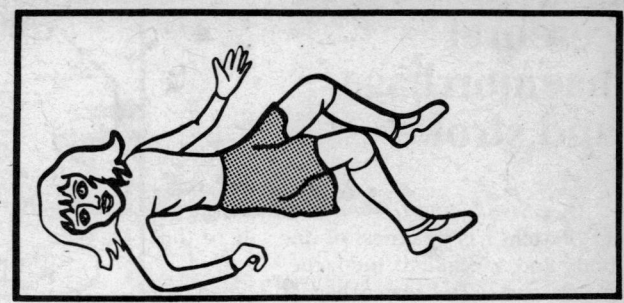

1   The commonest type of fit is *epilepsy*, where there will be purposeless movement of the arms and legs, possibly foaming at the mouth, and maybe biting of the tongue. (See *epilepsy*.) The patient must be prevented from harming himself while the fit is in progress, i.e. make sure he is not near a fire or sharp objects. When the fit is over put him in the coma/recovery position.

2   Behaviour of people who have epileptiform seizures varies greatly. Some come round quickly, others will go to sleep. Make sure, when the fit is over, that they are comfortable and that their airway is not obstructed. Do not force hard objects between the teeth to protect the tongue. Most people who have epileptiform seizures would rather have a bitten tongue than broken teeth.

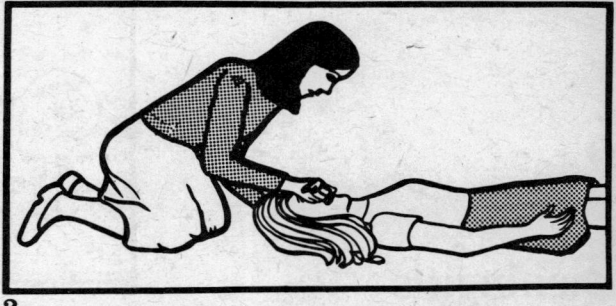

diabetic coma

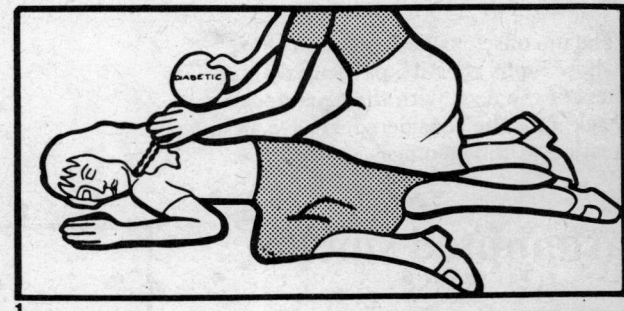

1 and 2   If you suspect diabetic coma look for a diabetic disc, or sugar lumps in the pocket and needle marks. In these days of drug addiction one would have to be aware of drug overdosage with signs of self injection for possible alternative diagnosis to diabetes.

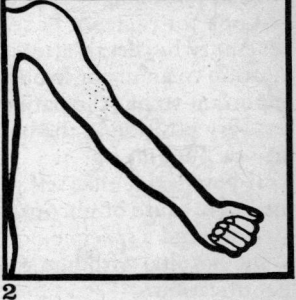

cerebral haemorrhage and stroke

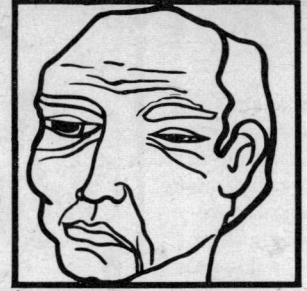

1

(See *Stroke* and *Cerebral Haemorrhage*.)
1   Patient has weakness of one side of the body and one side of the face.
2   Patient with haemorrhage in coma/recovery position.

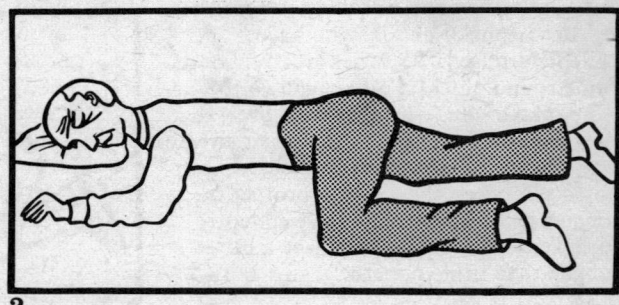

2

meningitis

The unconscious patient who is hot, whose limbs are stiff, particularly stiffness of the neck with the neck drawn back, must be considered to have an infection of the meninges.

attempted suicide

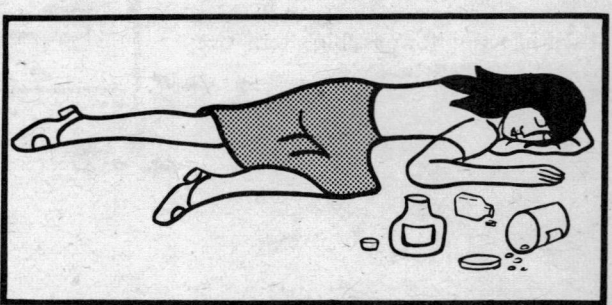

1

(Self poisoning — see *Poisoning*.)
1   Look for evidence of self poisoning, i.e. empty bottles, scattered pills, in close location to an unconscious patient. It is important to put the patient in the coma/recovery position as the intake of drugs may be building up.

If you decide that self poisoning is the likely cause of unconsciousness in the patient, send a specimen of pills or vomit to the hospital with him to help in their identification.

gaseous poisoning causing unconsciousness

(See *Poisoning*.)
1   Do not forget to remove immediately from gas-filled surroundings and then commence resuscitation (see *Resuscitation*).

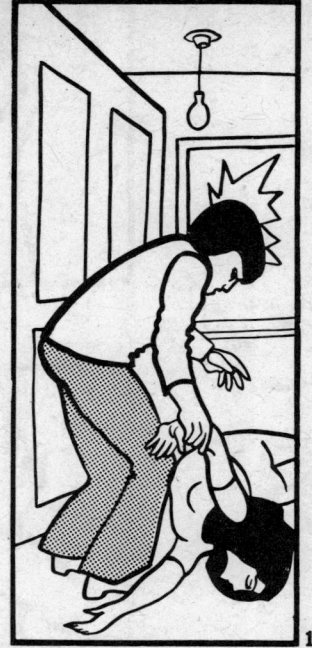

alcohol

1   Suspect alcohol being the cause of unconsciousness if the patient has an aroma of alcohol or is in the situation where alcohol is being consumed in large quantities. Look out for secondary causes, such as head injuries, and be careful that this is not a diabetic coma or a cerebral haemorrhage.

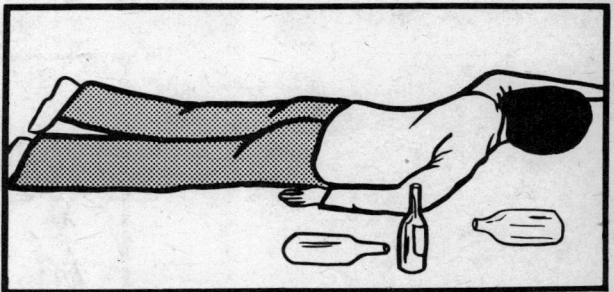

Footnote: The general principle of treatment for all unconscious patients is the same. Put them in the coma/recovery position.

Assess, on the guide lines laid down, the likely cause of unconsciousness. Seek immediate medical help, giving the information you have acquired by your assessment of the situation. Constantly attend the patient until medical help arrives, particularly his breathing, pulse rate and general colour and condition.

39

the arm

bleeding
of the fingers

1   A bleeding finger.
2   Hold the arm up vertically and apply pressure round the wrist to reduce the blood flow to the fingers.
3   Apply direct, firm pressure to the bleeding fingers and apply pad.
4   A pad bandage applied to bleeding area.
5   A complete bandaged finger.

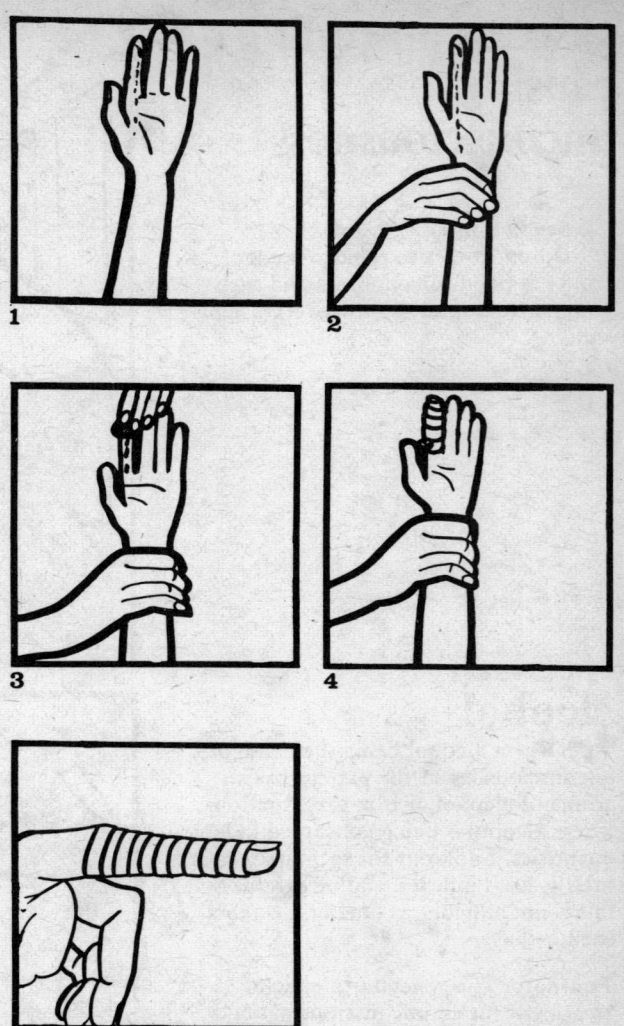

bleeding from the palm of the hand

1   Bleeding from the palm of the hand may be severe as several blood vessels are involved. Raise the limb where possible, and apply direct pressure to the wound.
2   Reduce the blood flow by gripping round the wrist. Cover the wound with a dressing.
3   Make a firm pad and put dressing in pad in palm of hand. Instruct the patient to make a fist over the pad.
4 to 7   Bandage the fist firmly with either a folded triangular bandage or an ordinary cotton bandage, tying the fingers down. The end of the bandage should be crossed under the base of the thumb (5). Support the limb with a sling.

continued overleaf

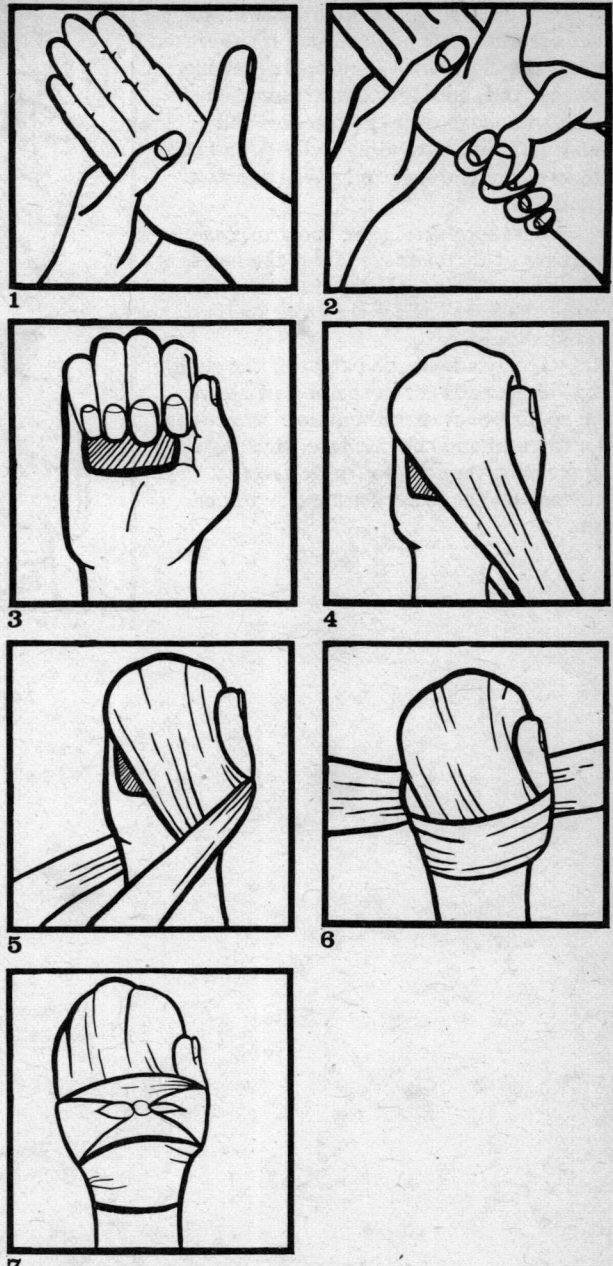

41

8   For supporting injured arm with sling, the forearm of the injured side is supported across the chest with the fingers pointing towards the shoulder of the sound side. Place a bandage over the forearm and hand, its point extending well beyond the elbow with its upper end over the sound shoulder.

9   Whilst supporting the forearm, ease the base of the bandage under the hand, forearm and elbow. Carry the lower end round the back, under the front of the sound shoulder.

10   Gently adjust the height of the sling and tie the ends off in the hollow above the collar bone, tuck the point in between the forearm and the bandage, finish off by securing the fold so formed to the bandage on the lower part of the upper arm.

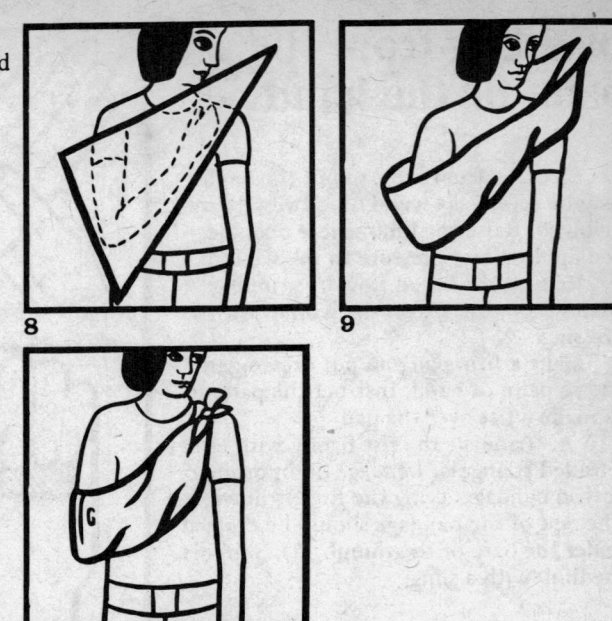

8

9

10

bleeding from the back of the hand

1 A cut on the back of the hand.
2 Elevate the limb, apply pressure round the wrist.
3 Apply direct pressure to wound, pad and bandage, keeping the limb elevated and cover with a hand bandage. Where the laceration is a long one and cannot be contained by the dressing, pinch the sides of the cut together.
4 The start of a sequence of bandages to enclose the hand for all injuries of the hand. The hand is laid on the base of a triangular bandage and the apex brought over.
5 The ends of the bandages are brought round to the front of the hand and crossed.
6 The bandage is then tied at the back of the wrist.
7 The completed bandage, with the tail of bandage tucked in.

continued overleaf

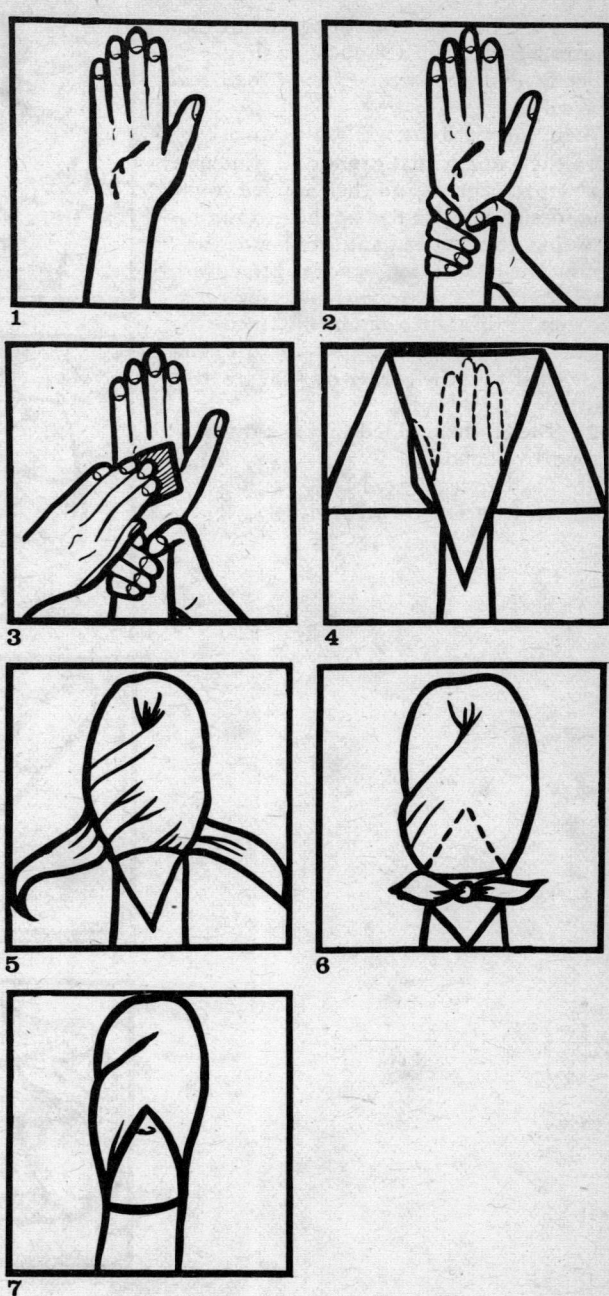

43

8 to 10   The sequence of procedures for putting the arm in a supportive sling. (See *Bleeding from the Palm of the Hand,* page 41.)

Where there are foreign bodies stuck into the wounds that cannot be removed, a ring pad is made and then applied round the foreign body, a pad applied to the dressing, the ring pad and pad bandaged round the hand, hand bandaged to cover the hand, and the arm put in a sling till further medical help can be obtained.

First fold the corner of a square of cloth.

11   First fold the corner of a square of cloth.

12   The cloth is folded to make thick, supportive bandage.

13   The bandage is twisted . . .

14   . . . into a circle on itself.

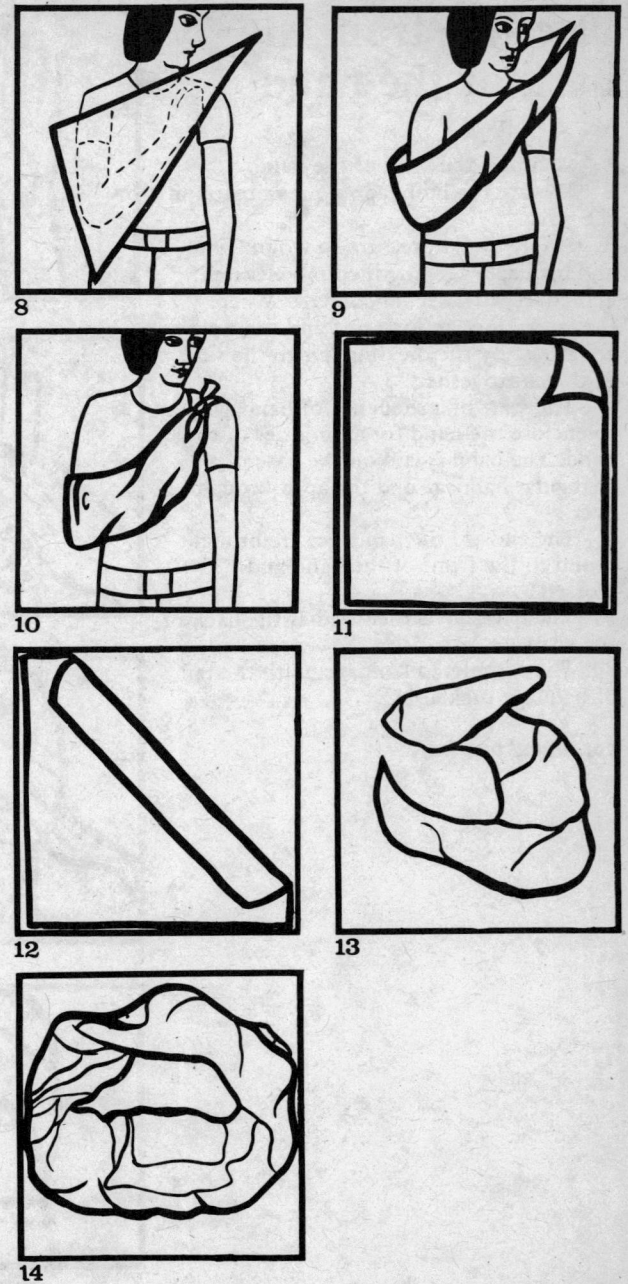

144

15 Ring pad being applied round foreign body in hand.
16 Pad being placed over ring pad.
17 Hand bandage being applied.
Hand is placed along the base of triangular bandage with apex pulled over wrist.
18 The opposite ends of the base of the triangle are brought round wrist.
19 The ends of the base of the triangle are tied at back of wrist.
20 The completed bandage.

continued overleaf

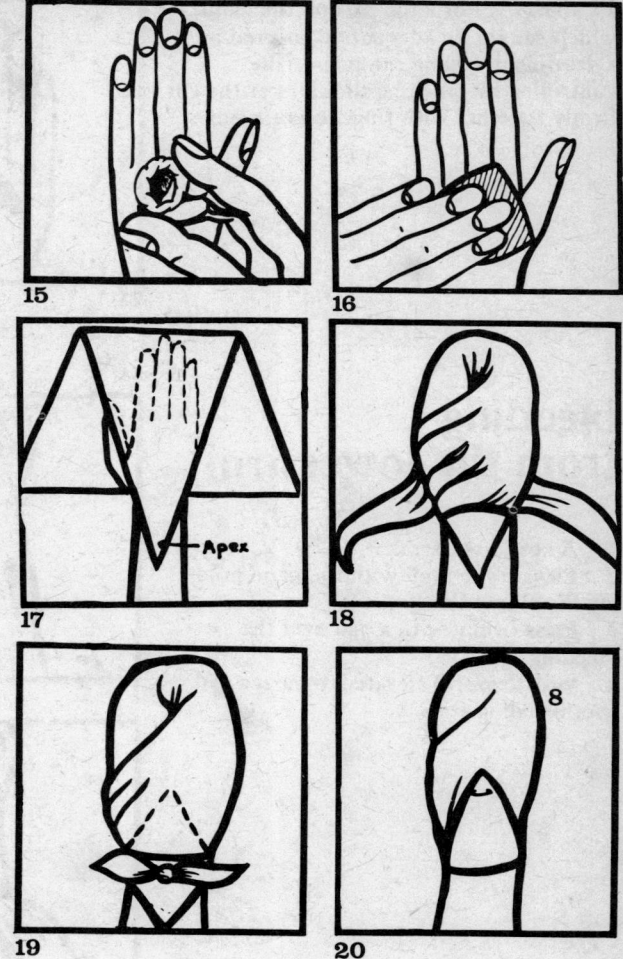

21 and 22 For large cuts on the hand which cannot be adequately covered by a dressing, bleeding can be initially controlled by pinching the sides of the cut firmly together with finger and thumb.

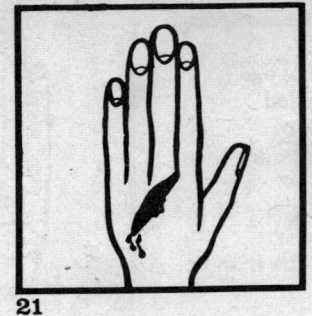

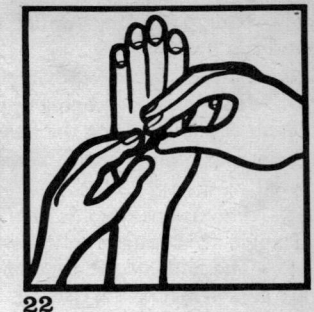

bleeding from the lower arm

1 A cut to the arm.
2 Elevate the limb with the hand holding the elbow firmly.
3 Press firmly with a pad over the bleeding area.
4 With arm still elevated, bandage pad over bleeding area.

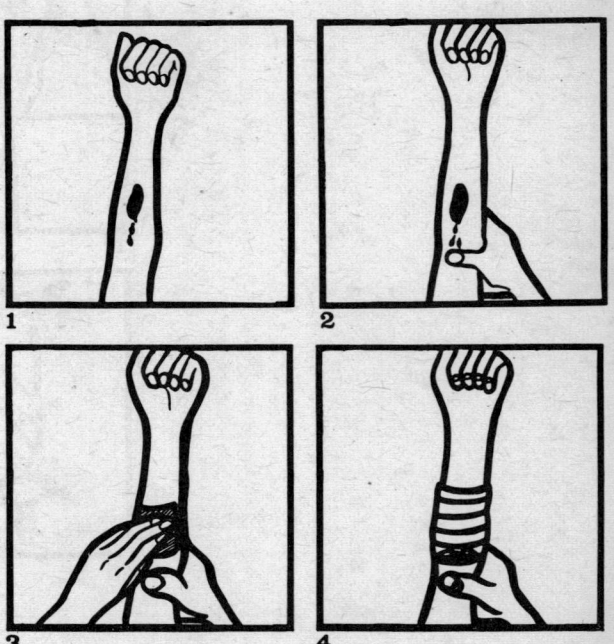

5   In circumstances where there is a foreign body in the wound, first make ring pad, then apply ring pad and pad to wound and bandage. If wound is a severe one, keep limb elevated.

6   Carry the lower end of the bandage round the back, under the front of the sound shoulder.

7   Tie the ends off in the hollow of the collar bone. Tuck the point in between the forearm and the bandage, secure the fold so formed to the bandage on the lower part of the upper arm.

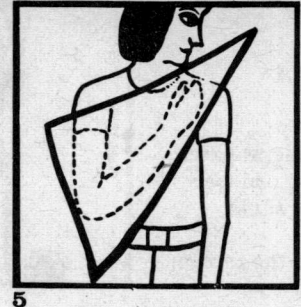

5

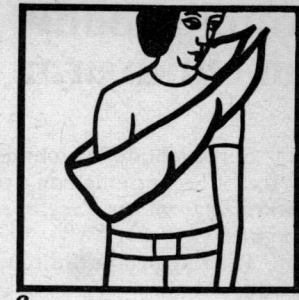

6

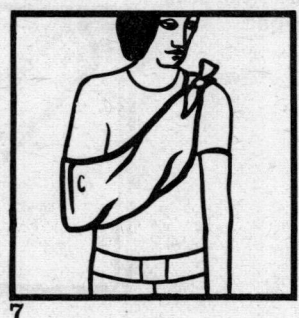

7

foreign body in cut in arm

1   Foreign body in wound. Elevate arm.
2 to 5   Steps in making a ring pad (see *Bleeding from the Back of the Hand*, page 43.)
6   The ring pad in situ round the foreign body.
7   Dressing pad being applied to the arm.
8   The bandaged pad in position.

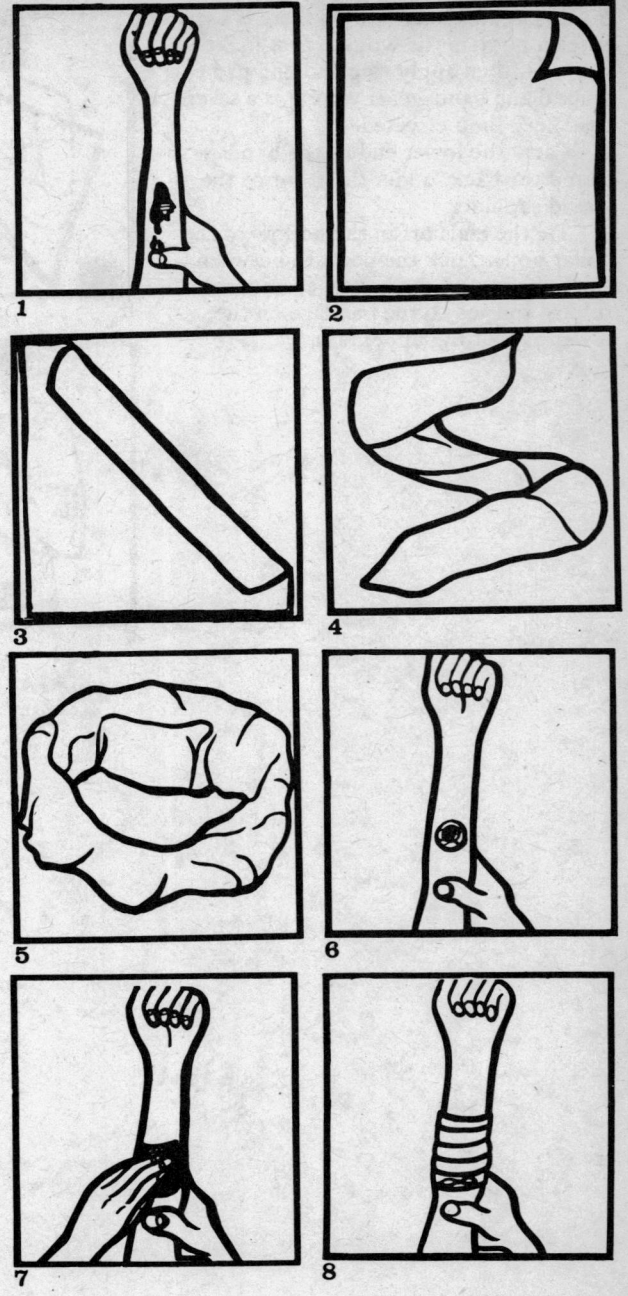

9 to 11 The sequence of movements for putting the arm in a sling (see *Bleeding from the Palm of the Hand*, page 41).

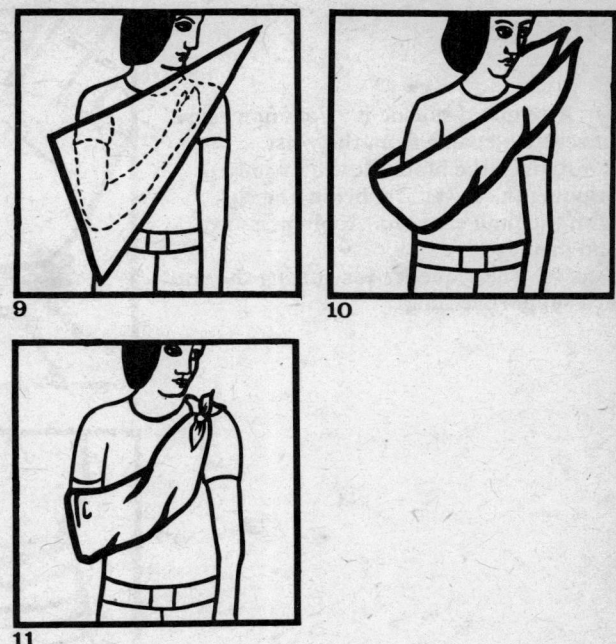

suicide

1   Attempted suicide is a common cause of severe bleeding from the wrist.
2   Reduce the blood flow by firmly gripping the lower arm below the cut, with the limb elevated. Apply pressure, and bandage.
3 to 5   The sequence for putting the arm in a supportive sling.

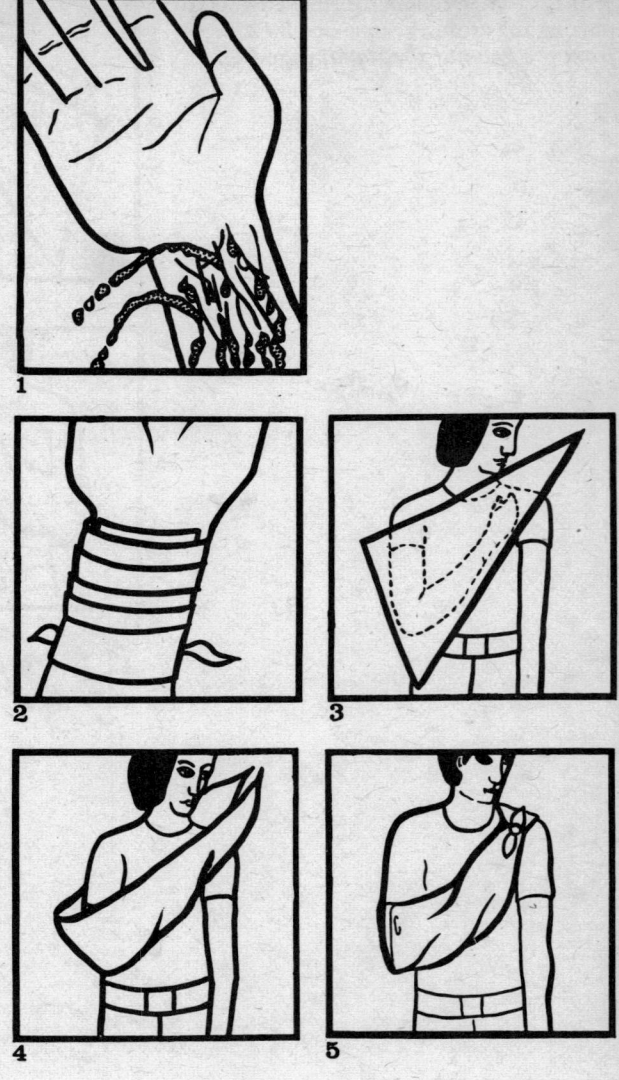

bleeding from the upper arm

1   A cut to the upper arm.
2   Where possible, elevate the arm above the head, probably with resting hand on top of head. Apply pressure between the cut and the shoulder to reduce the blood flow.
3   Apply pad to cut with firm pressure.
4   Bandage pad in situ. Depending on the severity of the cut, the arm may or may not be put in a sling.
5   A foreign body in cut on upper arm.
6 to 9   Making ring pad to put round foreign body. (See *Bleeding from the Back of the Hand*.)

continued overleaf

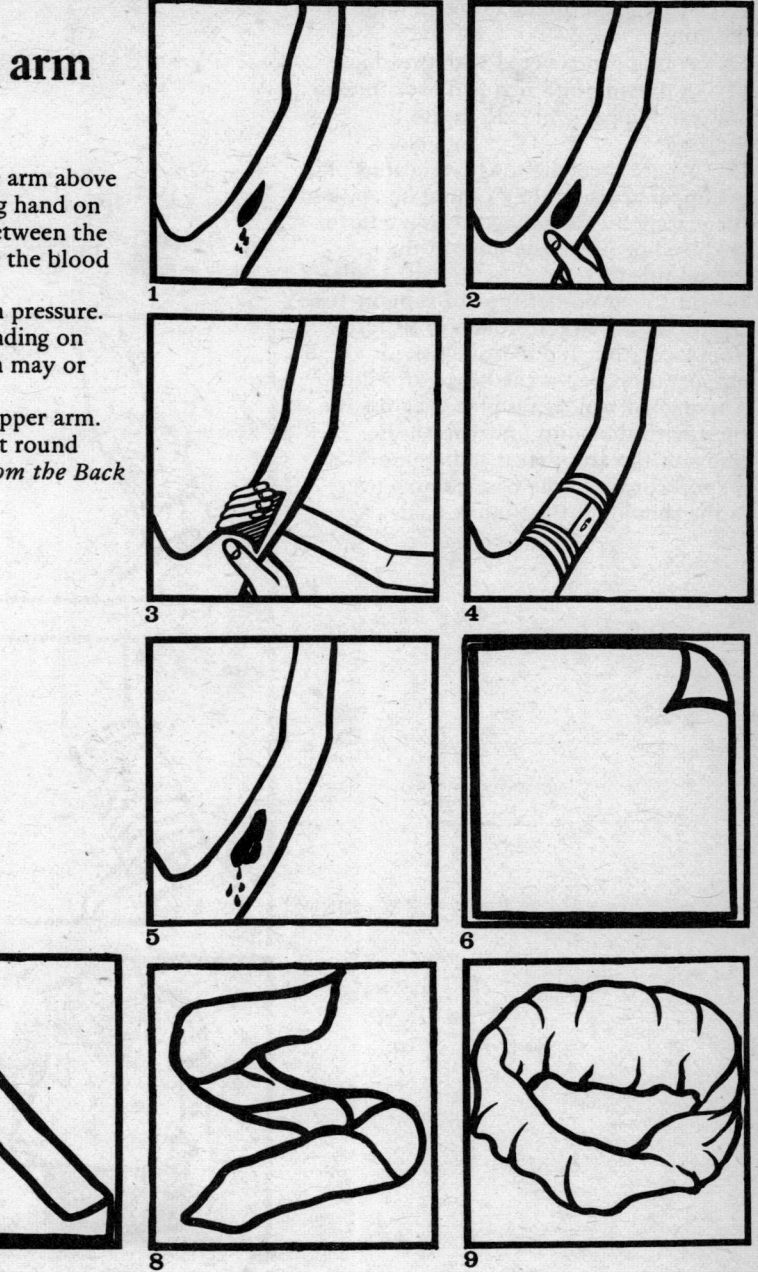

10   A ring pad round a foreign body in the arm.

11   A ring pad covered with dressing.

12   A dressing and ring pad over foreign body and upper arm held in situ by bandage.

13   Where there are long lacerations of the upper arm and they cannot be covered adequately by a dressing, to help control the bleeding pinch the sides of the wound together.

14 and 15   Another type of support for an arm that is either broken or suffering from laceration and bleeding where support is needed is the broad arm sling. A triangular bandage is placed across the chest with the point underneath the elbow of the arm that is to be supported, the top corner of the base coming over to the shoulder of the injured side.

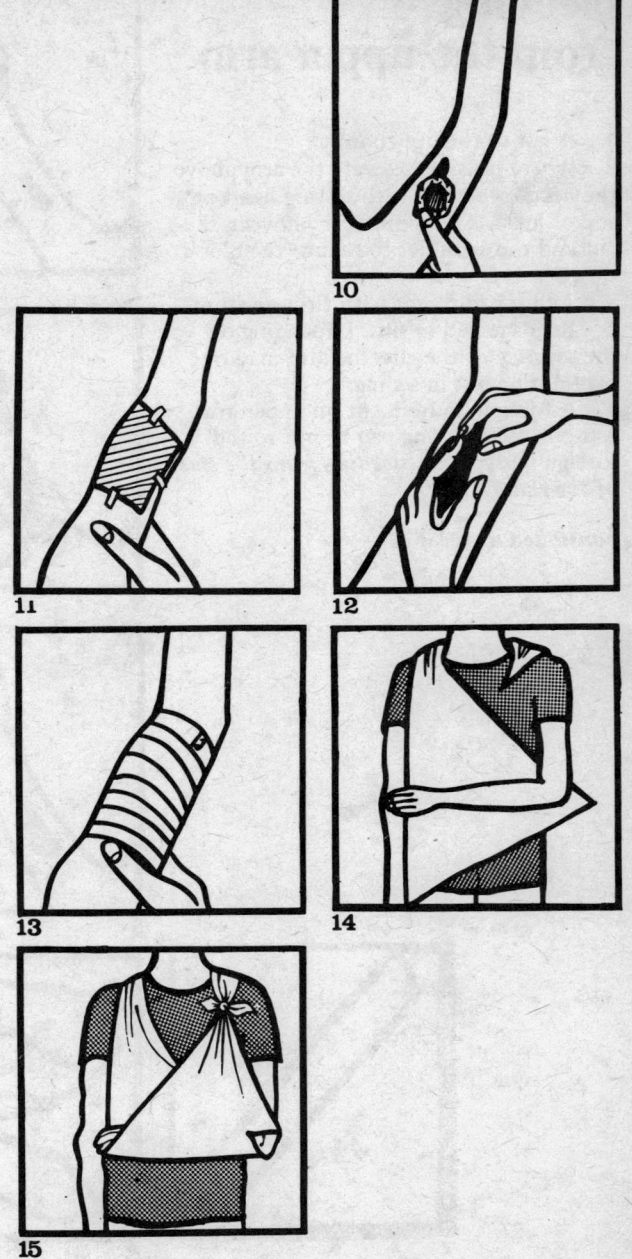

bleeding from amputations

1 An amputated finger.
2 Elevate the limb, tie constricting tape round the lower end of the finger firmly enough to stop the flow of blood; apply firm dressing to cut end, apply pressure at wrist, bandage pressure pad to top of bleeding end, support hand with wrist elevated in an arm sling. Hospitalisation will be required.
3 With the wrist firmly gripped by your hand apply a pad to the end of the amputation, with tape to reduce blood flow.
4 Bandage pad on to finger and remove restricting tape, still supporting at wrist.
5 Lay triangular bandage across injured arm.
6 Carry the lower end round the back, under the front of the sound shoulder.
7 Tie the ends off in the hollow of the collar bone. Tuck the point in between the forearm and the bandage, secure the fold so formed to the bandage on the lower part of the upper arm.

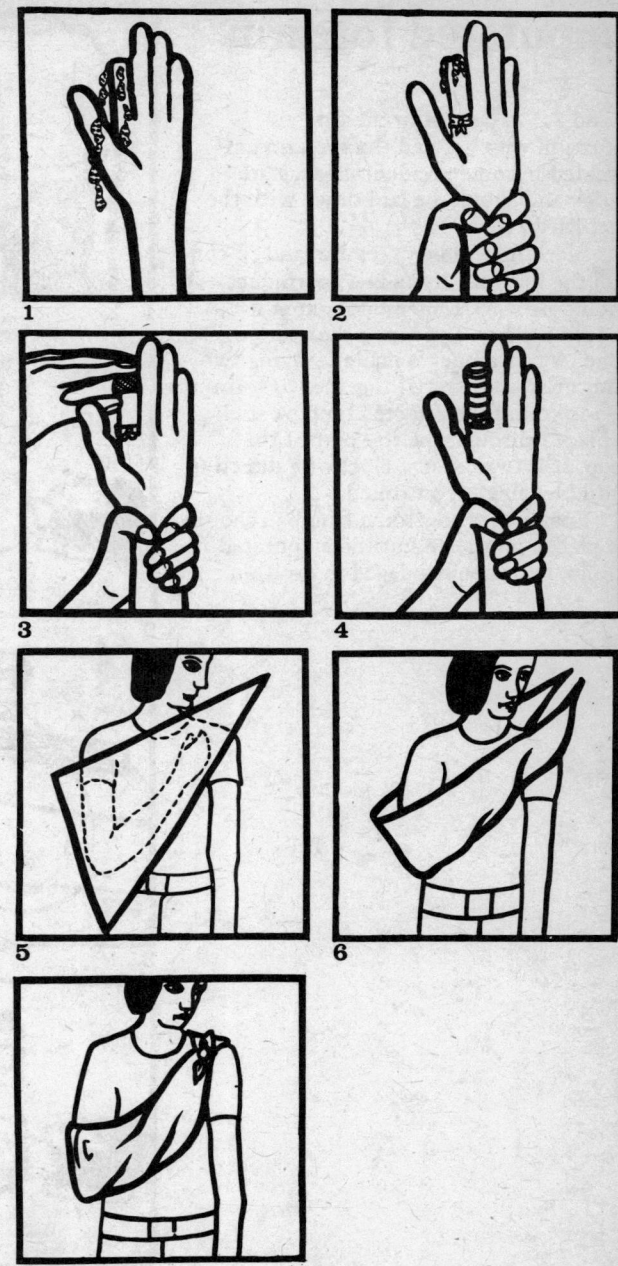

amputated forearm

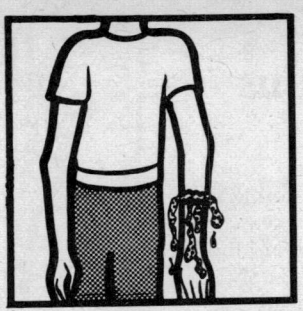

1 and 2 A patient in the first aid situation who has had the forearm amputated in some accident is in a state of shock and should be laid down with the limb elevated.

3 Bleeding will be excessive, and to control the bleeding initially a tourniquet should be used, remembering that it should be kept on for the shortest possible time. A tourniquet is made by tying two ends of stout material together to form a loop round the affected limb. A stick is placed through the top part of the loop. It is twisted in a clockwise direction until bleeding is controlled.

4 For further control, a firm pad should be placed on the end of the amputated stump, and then bandaged in position.

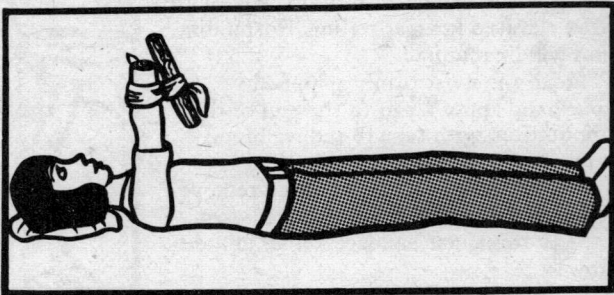

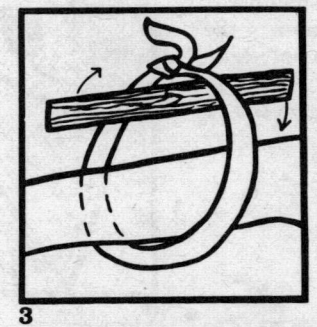

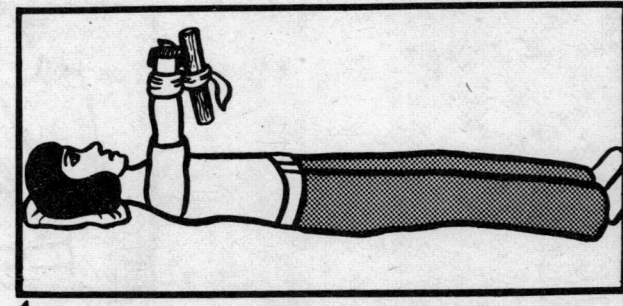

5 and 6   The pad is held in position by firm bandaging to and fro across the stump, starting and finishing well below the amputation site. This is then anchored by further bandaging *around* the stump.

7   Once the bandage is firmly in place, the tourniquet should slowly be released to see if bleeding is controlled. If bleeding is not controlled by the dressing, the tourniquet should be slowly released for 1 minute every 20 minutes and reapplied until expert medical attention has been sought.

8 to 10   After completion of dressing and arrest of bleeding the arm should be supported in a sling for transporting the patient.

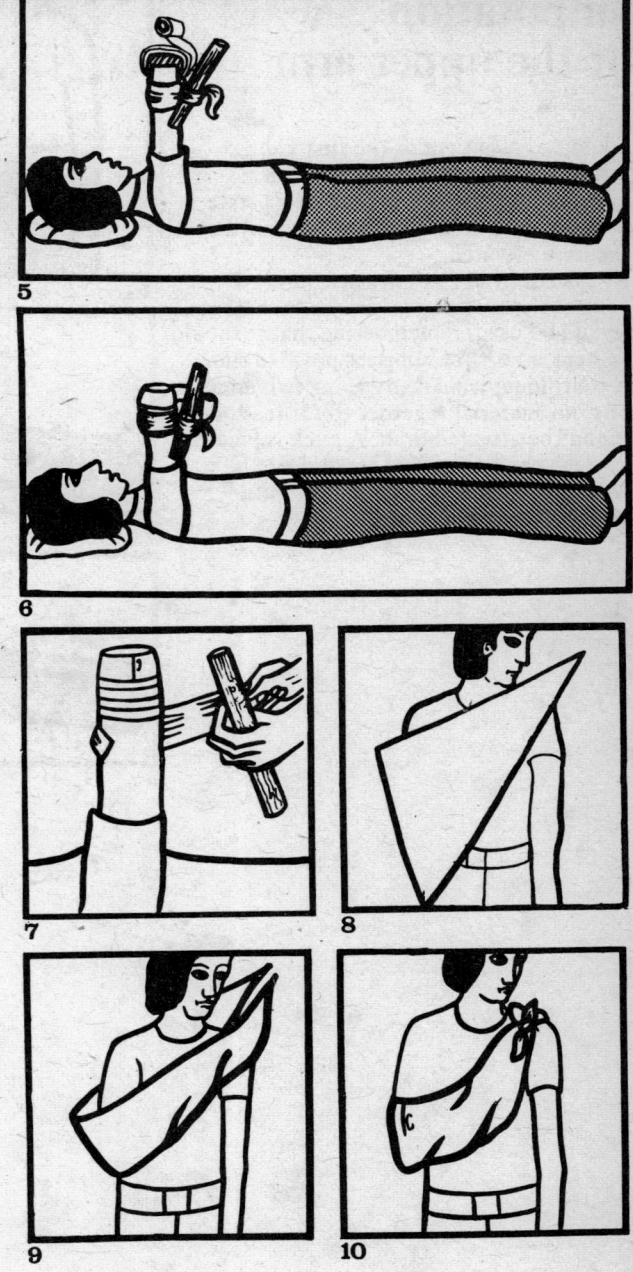

amputation
of the upper arm

1 and 2   A patient in the first aid
situation who has had the upper arm
amputated in some accident is in a state
of shock and should be laid down with
the limb elevated.
3   Bleeding will be excessive, and to
control the bleeding initially a tourniquet
should be used, remembering that it should
be kept on for the shortest possible time.
A tourniquet is made by tying two ends
of stout material together to form a loop
round the affected limb. A stick is placed
through the top part of the loop. It is
twisted in a clockwise direction until
bleeding is controlled.

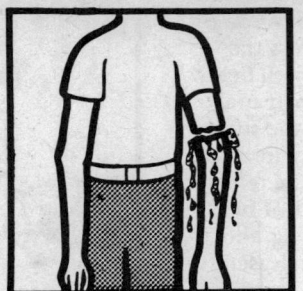
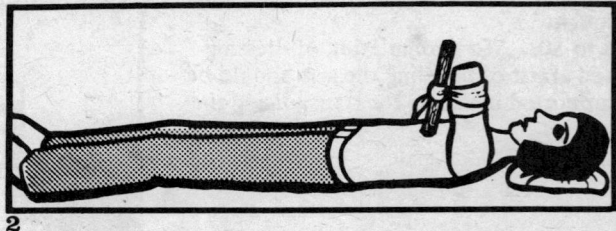
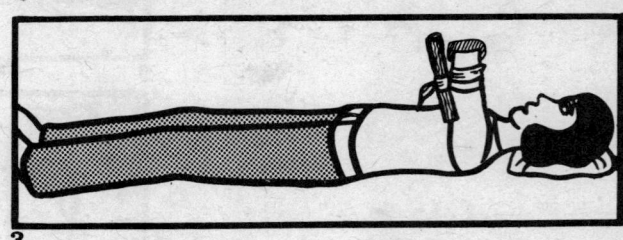

4 For further control, a firm pad should be placed on the end of the amputated stump, and then bandaged in position.

5 The pad is held in position by firm bandaging to and fro across the stump, starting and finishing well below the amputation site. This is then anchored by further bandaging *around* the stump.

6 Once the bandage is firmly in place, the tourniquet should be slowly released to see if bleeding is controlled. If bleeding is not controlled by the dressing, the tourniquet should be slowly released for 1 minute every 20 minutes and reapplied until expert medical attention has been sought.

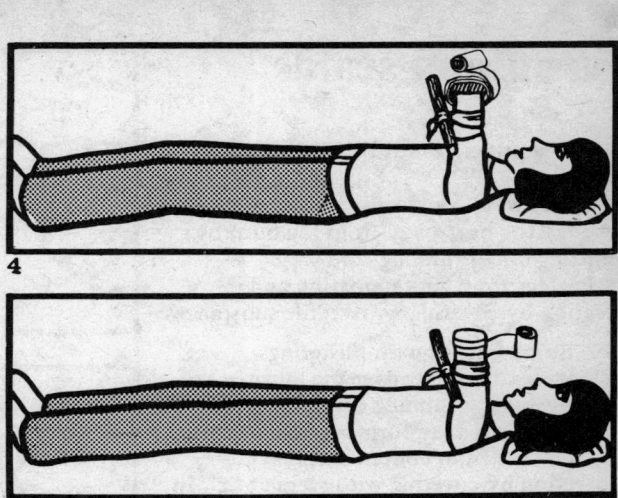

4

5

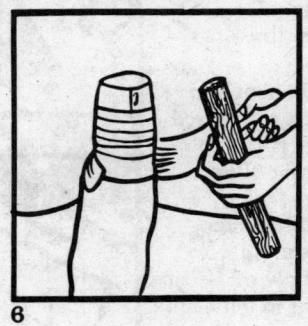

6

burns and scalds

General principles for treatment for burns are:
- Take away from heat.
- Take the heat away from the burn by putting under running cold water.
- Protect from contamination and infection by covering with sterile substances.

1   Burnt fingers, with blisterings.
2   Pour cold water over the burnt area or put under a running cold tap. Do not prick blisters, they form an ideal dressing.
3   Protect from contamination and infection by covering with sterile or clean material. If possible cover with paraffin gauze as this is the ideal dressing. Do not put on oils, butter or any other dressings.
4   Fingers can then be bandaged.
5   Where the hand is severely burnt and there is swelling, the arm is best supported in a sling. A triangular bandage is laid across chest to make a supportive sling for transporting patient.
6   Carry the lower end round the back, under the front of the sound shoulder.
7   Tie the ends off in the hollow of the collar bone. Tuck the point in between the forearm and the bandage, secure the fold so formed to the bandage on the lower part of the upper arm.

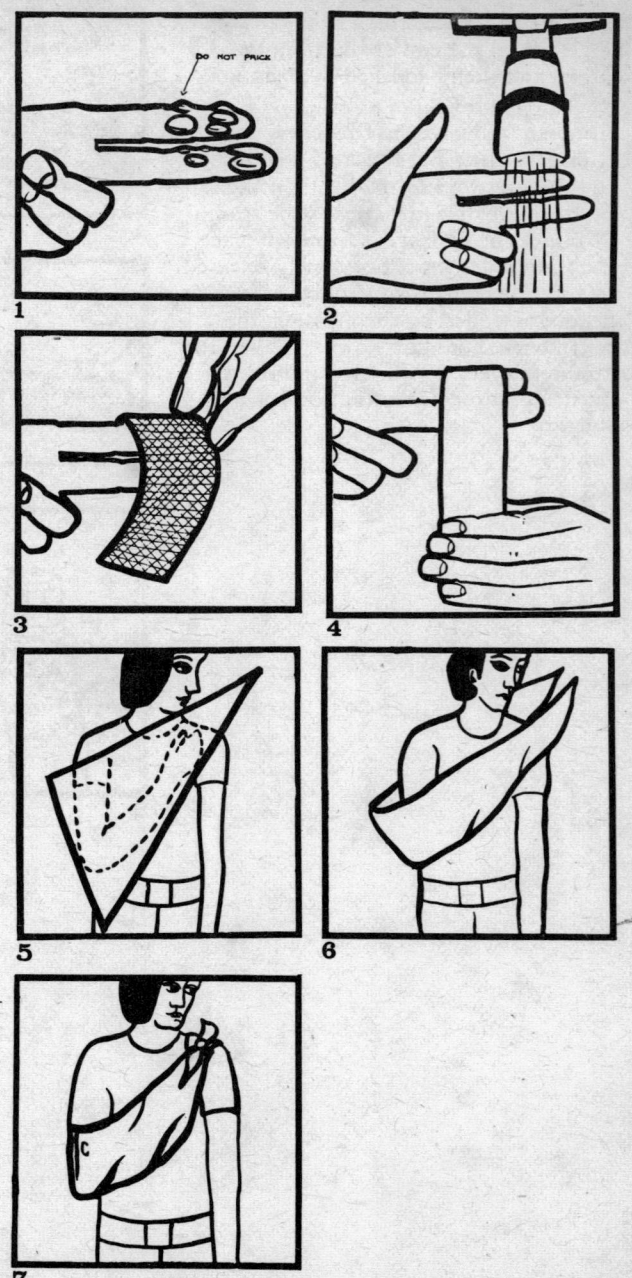

8   A large burn to the back of the hand.
9   For large burns, put the hand under a running cold tap for 5 to 10 minutes, or pour cold water from a jug over it.
10   When possible cover the burnt area with paraffin gauze, or cover the whole area with clean or sterile material.
11   The whole hand can be adequately covered by a triangular bandage in the form of a hand bandage. Place the palm of the hand over a triangular bandage or triangle of cloth, bringing the point over to the back of the wrist.
12   Bring the two points of the base of the triangle round to the back of the wrist, cross them and bring to the front to tie.
13 and 14   Tie on the front of the wrist and bring the protruding point of the triangle and pin to the back of the bandage.

continued overleaf

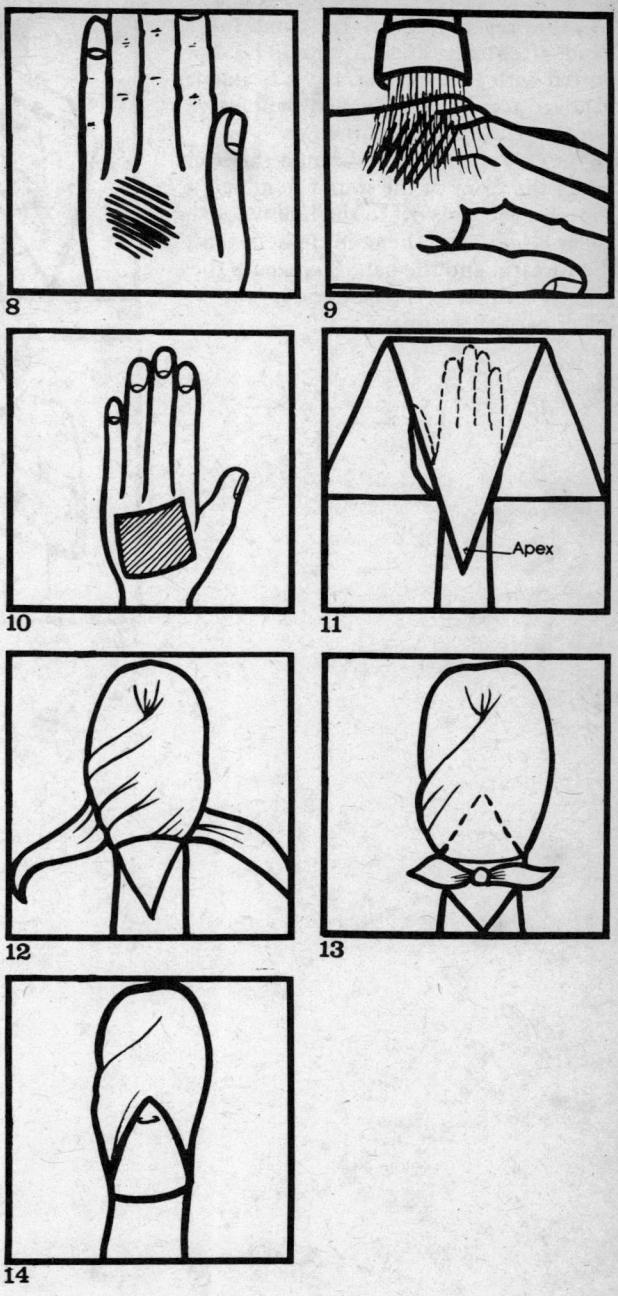

59

15 For severe burns to the hand, the hand, after being dressed, should be supported with an arm sling. Lay a triangular bandage across chest to make supportive sling for transporting patient.

16 Carry the lower end round the back under the front of the sound shoulder.

17 Tie the ends off in the hollow of the collar bone. Tuck the point in between the forearm and the bandage, secure the fold so formed to the bandage on the lower part of the upper arm.

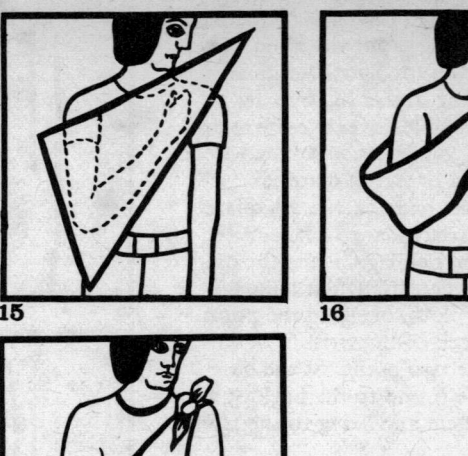

15

16

17

small burns to the arm

1 A small blistery burn to the forearm.
2 Pour water over the burn for 5 to 10 minutes.
3 If possible, cover with paraffin gauze and cover with sterile or clean material.
In the case of very small burns, clothing can be washed or removed from them.
Do not burst any blisters that are present, they are the best dressing a burn can have.
4 A large piece of material as a dressing can be applied to the burn.
5 and 6 Loosely bandage the covering to the arm.

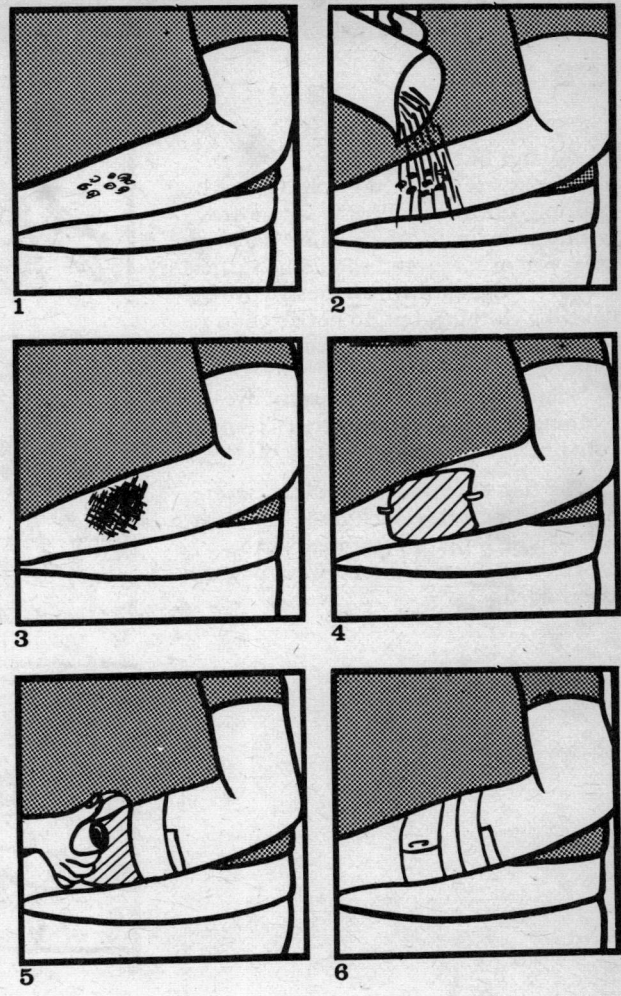

severe burns to the arm

1   A large burn to the arm.
2   For severe burns to the arm, treat by pouring cold water over the whole area burnt, including clothing. If no tap available, five or six jugsful should be sufficient.
3 and 4   Cut through any restrictive or covering clothing, but do not attempt to pick off clothing that has become fused with the burn.
5   Place cooled arm, with restrictive clothing loosened, in protective clean container, for example a pillow case.

The first aider must remember severe burns of any sort, even limited to one arm, will require hospital treatment as the depth of the burn cannot always be easily ascertained.

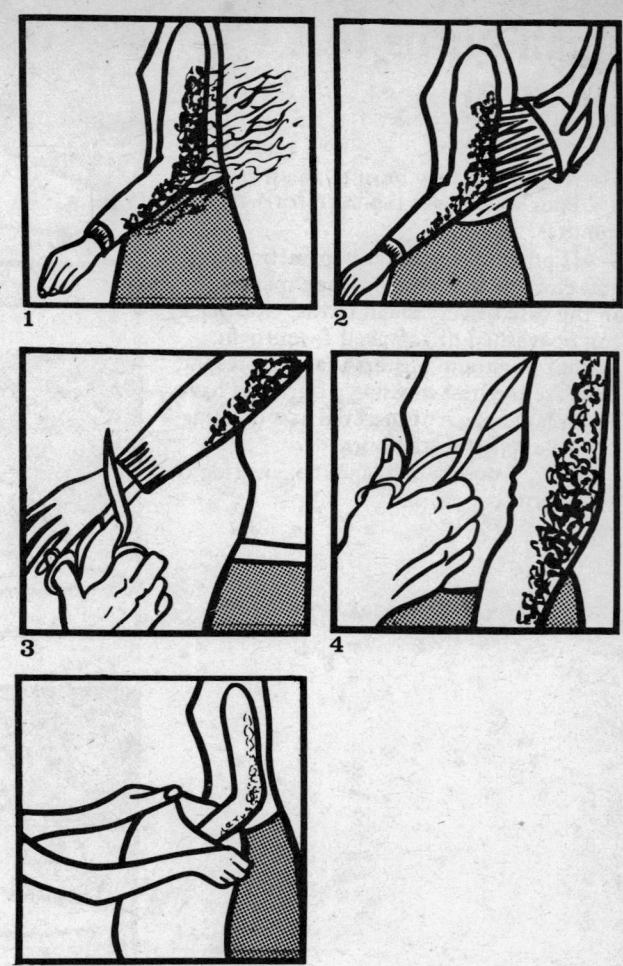

burns and cuts to the shoulder

For burns or cuts and abrasions to the shoulders, having cleaned and disinfected and put on either a pad over a cut or a paraffin gauze dressing for a burn, a shoulder bandage will keep the dressing in position.

1   The shoulder bandage is made from a triangular bandage or triangular piece of cloth. Lay the point of the bandage on the shoulder with the point towards the ear.
2 and 3   Take the two lower ends and cross them on the inside of the arm and bring to the outside, and tie.
4 and 5   A complete triangular bandage will help to prevent the arm swelling, with top of shoulder being tucked in.

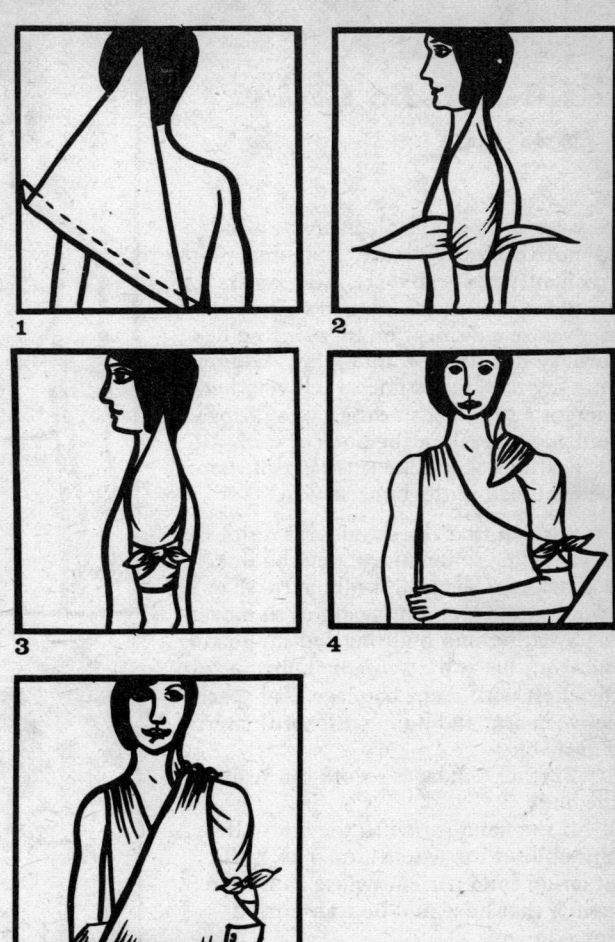

breaks and dislocations of the shoulder

A dislocation is a displacement of one or more bones at a joint. The joints most frequently dislocated are those of the shoulder, elbow, thumb and fingers. Recognise a dislocation by pain and deformity in a limb or limb joint. Without an x-ray it is impossible to tell whether there is a simple dislocation or a dislocation and a break in the bone as well. All dislocations should be treated as if there were a break in the bone as well.

1 Suspect that the shoulder is dislocated if, following some injury, one shoulder is a different shape and silhouette than the other shoulder and it is painful to move.
2 Treat by immobilising and supporting the arm, that is by tying the upper arm to the chest with crepe bandage. Pad space between arm and body with soft material, if available.
3 Further bandages secure the arm to the body.
4 If the hand is tied to the body, this immobilises the whole arm. This is the situation for a patient whose condition is such that he would be transported lying down.

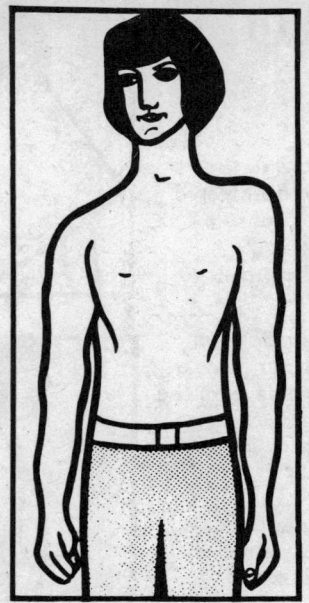

1

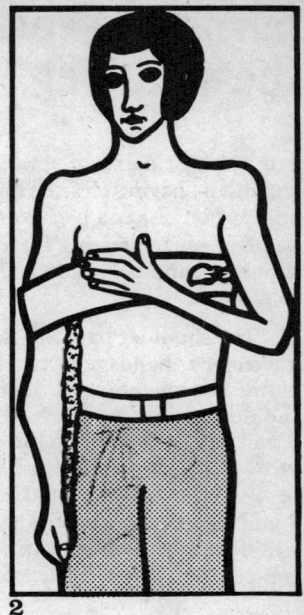

2

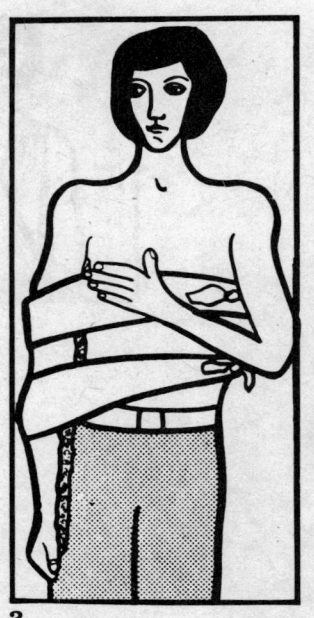

3

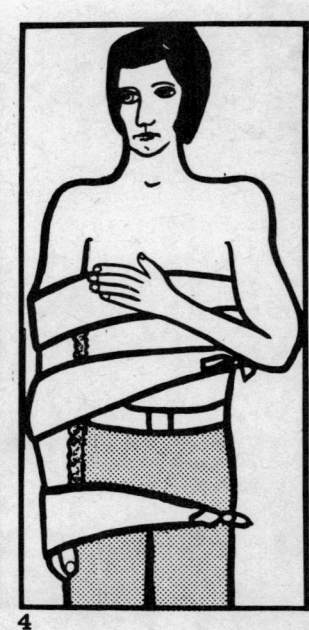

4

5 to 8 For the patient who can walk, if for example, this had been sustained after a games injury, splint the arm to the chest by tying two bandages round the upper arm to the chest, and then support the arm in a sling.

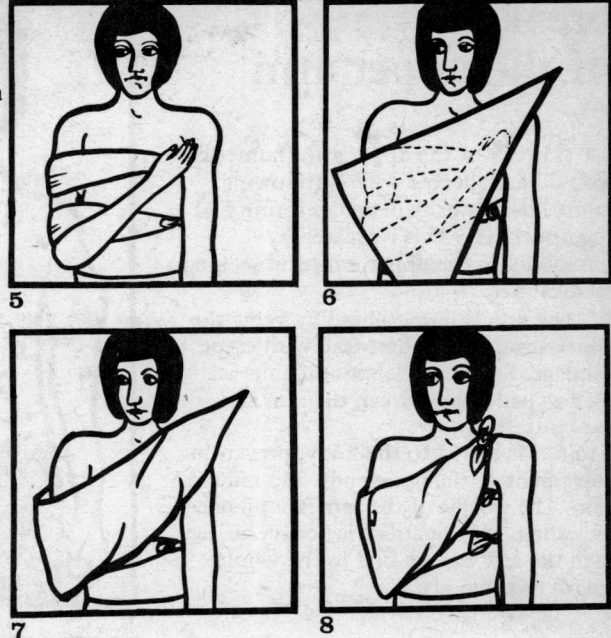

5

6

7

8

breaks
of the upper arm

1   A break of the upper arm (humerus) would be suspected where, following injury, there was pain and deformity of the upper arm. This is treated by immobilising the upper arm, and seeking medical help.

2   The arm is immobilised by tying the upper arm, to the chest wall with crepe bandage. Soft material, if available, is used as padding between the arm and the body.

3 to 6   It is tied to the body, preventing movement of the bone ends, and reducing pain. The weight of the arm is supported by a sling. If the patient is not on his feet, then the arm can be tied to the whole length of the body.

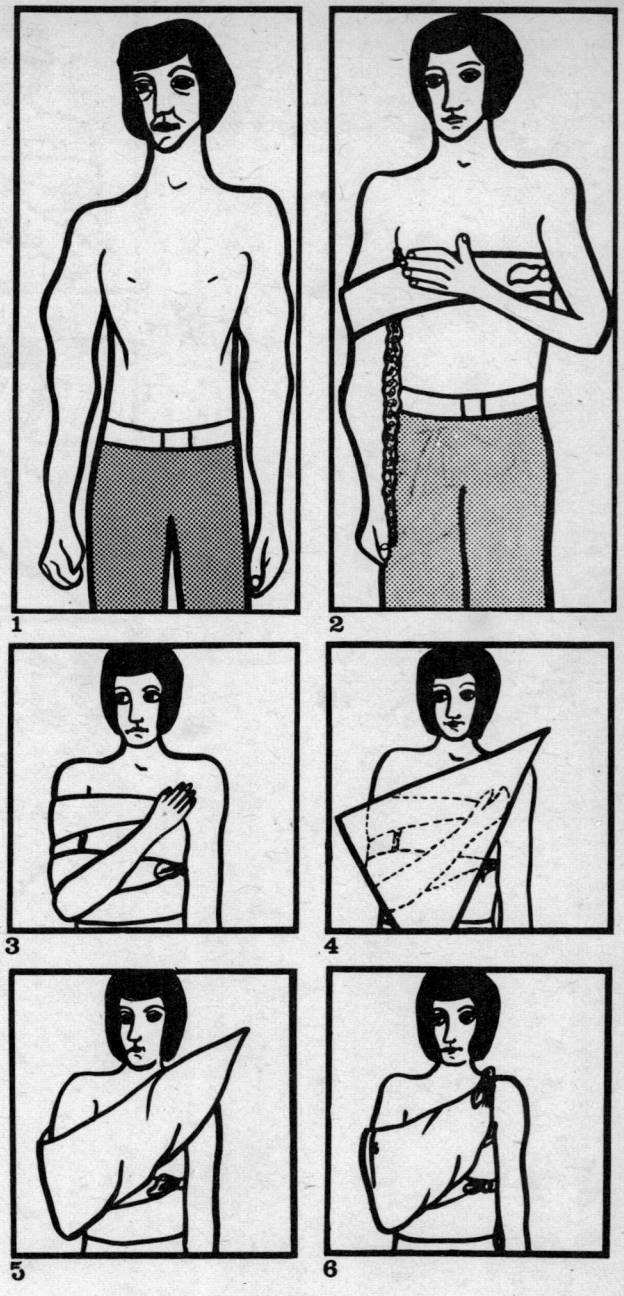

7 and 8 The arm is immobilised completely when the patient is not able to walk, the hand being secured to body to prevent further movement.

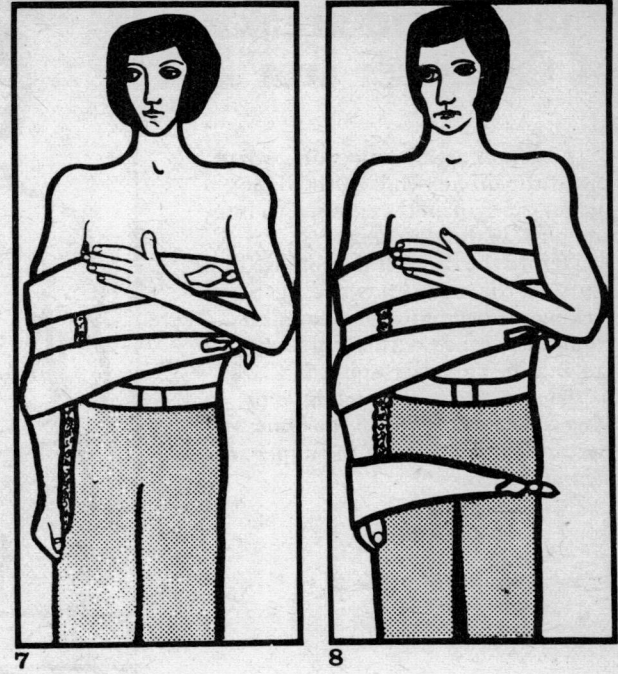

complicated breaks of the upper arm

1   A complicated break is one where one of the broken ends of the bone pierces the skin and is exposed to infection outside the skin area.

2   Before the break is immobilised, the injury on the arm wall where the bone is sticking through must be treated. It should be cleaned with disinfectant, a pad and firm bandage applied.

3   Then the arm is immobilised by tying to the chest wall in the same way that the simple break of the upper arm is immobilised.

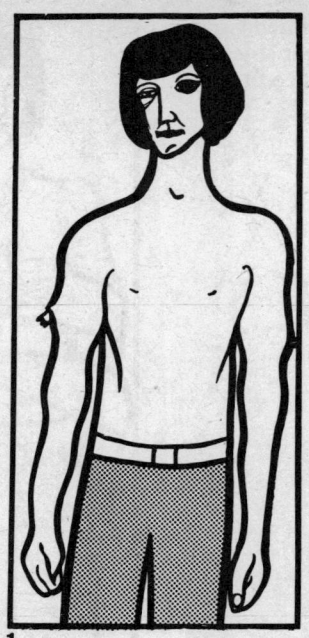
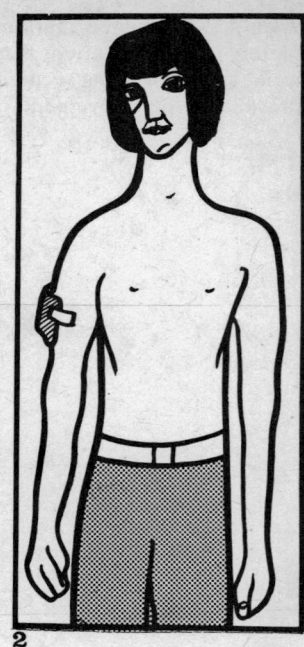
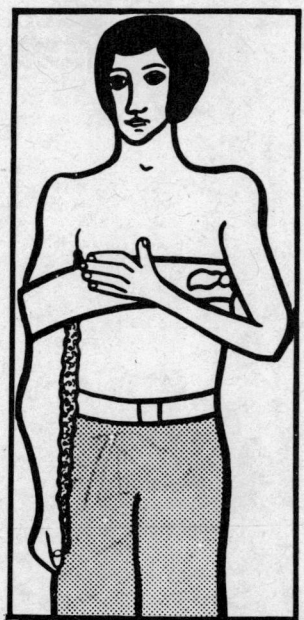

4   A second tie completes the fixing of the upper arm to the chest wall.

5   A triangular bandage is laid across the chest in the first stage of making a supportive sling for transporting the patient.

6   Carry the lower end round the back, and under the front of the sound shoulder.

7   Tie the ends off in the hollow of the collar bone. Tuck the point in between the forearm and the bandage, and secure the fold so formed to the bandage on the lower part of the upper arm.

8 and 9   Where the patient is not walking about, then the arm is splinted to the whole of the body, a bandage fixing the hand round the thighs.

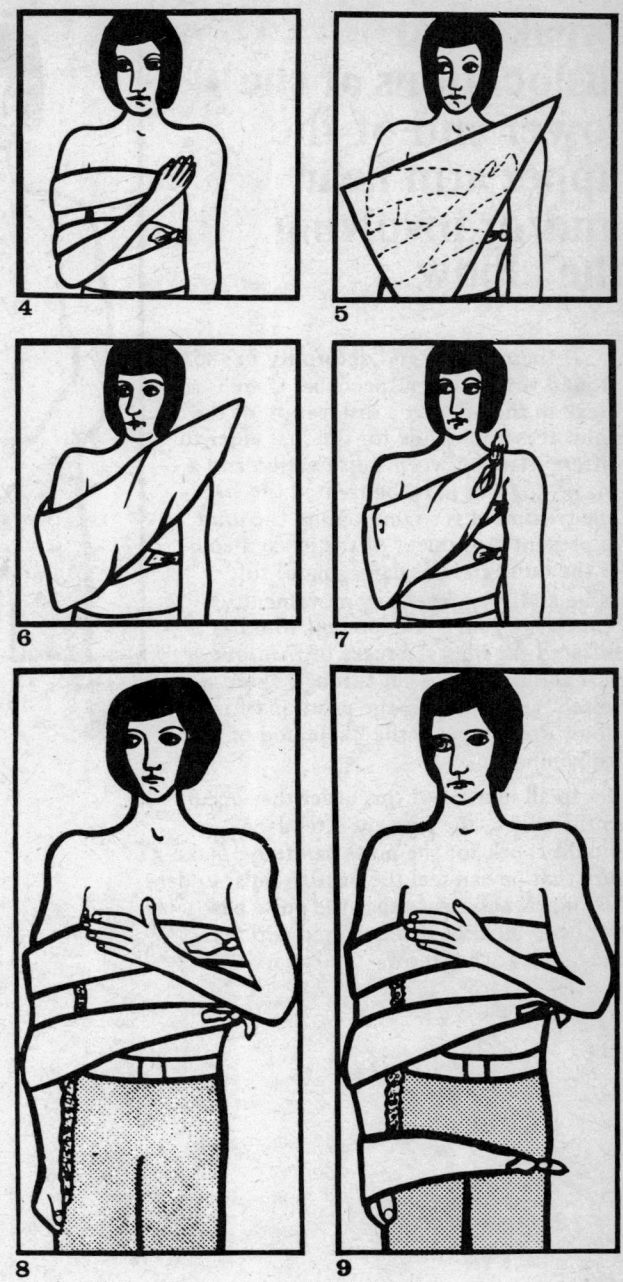

breaks and dislocations at the lower end of the upper arm near and/or involving the elbow

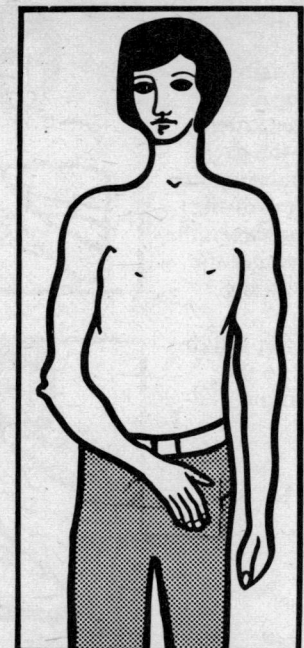

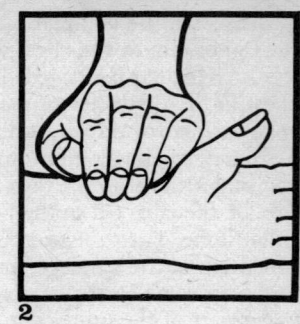

1   If there is pain and deformity in and around the elbow, suspect that there is a break in the bone or a dislocation of the joint. It is impossible for the first aider to differentiate between a dislocation and a break, so both must be treated the same. The treatment is to immobilise the joint to prevent movement of the broken ends of the bone and the damaging of soft tissue and, by preventing movement, reduce the pain to the patient who has suffered the injury. Breaks of the bone near the elbow can cut through blood vessels, and changing the position of the elbow does increase the likelihood of this happening.

2   In all injuries of this order that occur to the elbow, the first aid attendant should check for the pulse carefully, making sure that he can feel the beating pulse under his finger. Make sure that the pulse has not been blocked or interfered with by the break at the elbow.

3 to 6   Pad the elbow with soft material and immobilise it by splinting it to the body, tying bandages round the arm and the chest wall, waist and upper thighs. The arm should be kept at a slightly bent angle, the hand pointing to the groin. This immobilises the whole of the right upper limb. In no circumstances should there be any attempt to straighten the arm or put it back in shape in any way as this can lead to serious damage to blood vessels.

continued overleaf

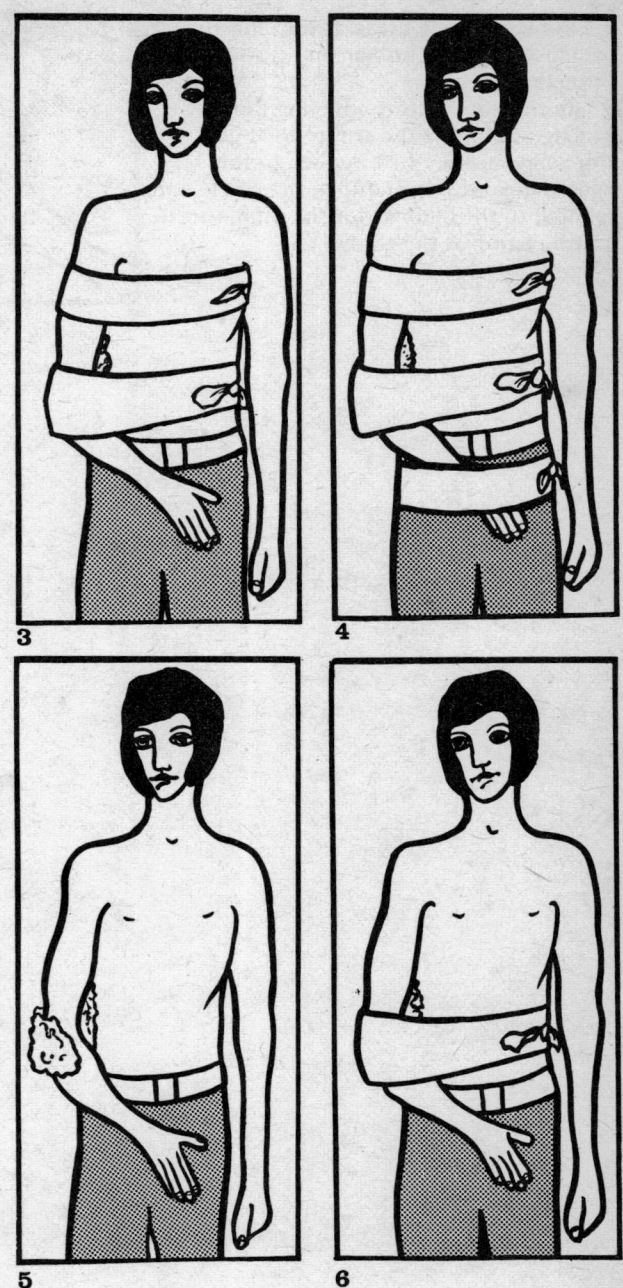

7 Sometimes the break at the elbow is complicated and a broken end is sticking through the skin.

8 In this case, before applying the bandages splinting the arm to the body, a dressing must be first applied to the injured area of skin and then the whole limb splinted to the body as for the simple break or dislocation at the elbow.

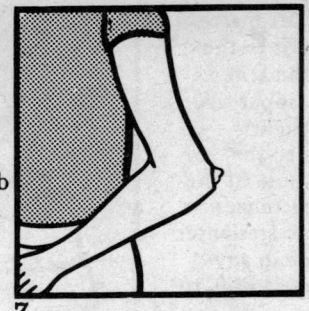 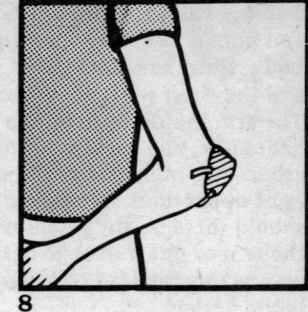

7

8

breaks of the lower arm between elbow and wrist

1 Recognise that the lower arm may be broken by the presence of deformity of the lower arm, and pain.

2 To prevent the broken ends of the bones doing damage inside the arm, and to reduce pain of the patient, splint the arm (in this case it cannot be tied to the body, so a piece of wood or a magazine, preferably padded, will suffice).

3 Lay the supported arm on the splint, pad, bandage the splint to the arm.

4 Support the arm in a wide triangular bandage. Spread the triangular bandage across the body, under the arm, pointing towards the injured arm.

5 Completion of the triangular bandage, with the lower point brought up to be tied over the injured shoulder.

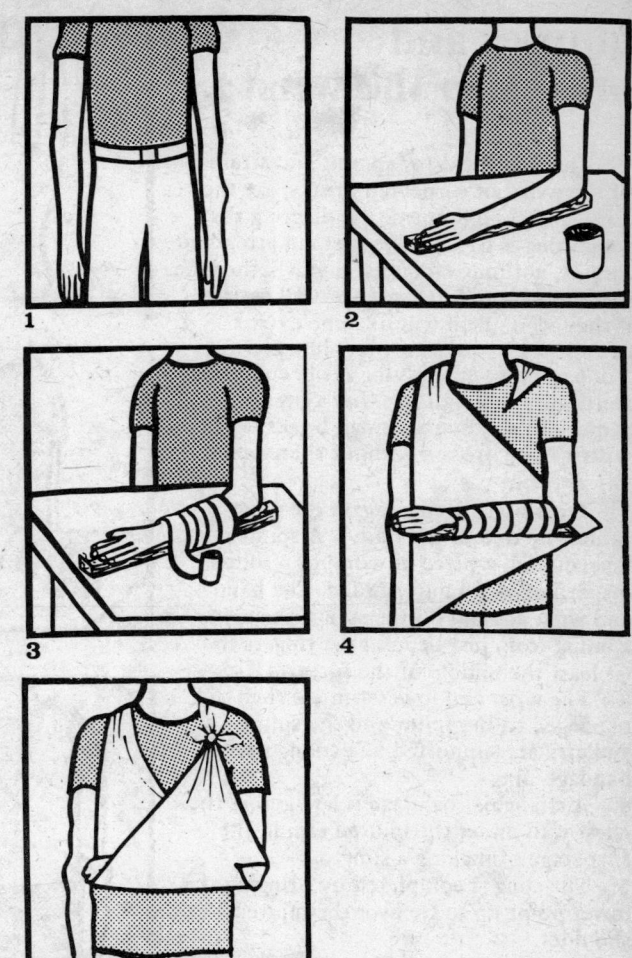

injuries and breaks to the wrist

1   The treatment for sprains and strains of the wrist, or suspected breaks, are the same, pain and deformity indicating that something is wrong. The first aid attendant cannot, without x-rays, decide whether the wrist is broken, but must treat all cases as if they were. Pain will to some extent be relieved by pouring on cold water for 5 or 6 minutes or applying a cold compress. Deformity will indicate that a break is more likely, but the small bones of the ; wrist can be broken without there being any deformity.

2   Treat by splinting (again the wrist cannot be tied to the body). A splint must be acquired, a piece of wood or a rolled magazine, preferably padded. The hand and wrist are laid on the splint, the splint coming from just beyond the fingers to at least the middle of the forearm.

3   The wrist and lower arm are then bandaged to the splint and the splint and arm are supported in a triangular bandage sling.

4   A triangular bandage is laid across the chest wall under the injured arm in the first stage of making a sling.

5   The sling is completed by bringing the lower point up to tie over the injured shoulder.

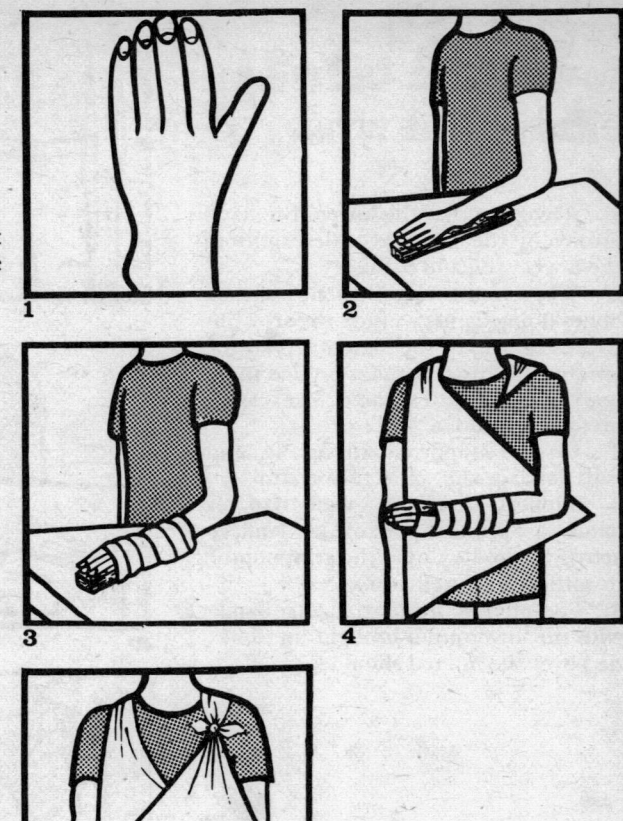

breaks and injuries to fingers

1 Fingers can be both broken and dislocated. It is very difficult for the first aid attendant to decide whether a dislocated finger is a simple dislocation or whether there is a break and a dislocation.

2 and 3 Support the injured part as best you can by packing and immobilising. Distorted finger positions, accompanied by pain following trauma, suggest breaks.

Pack the deformed hand with fingers clenched over soft material to restrict movement.

4 to 7 Cover with hand bandage.

continued overleaf

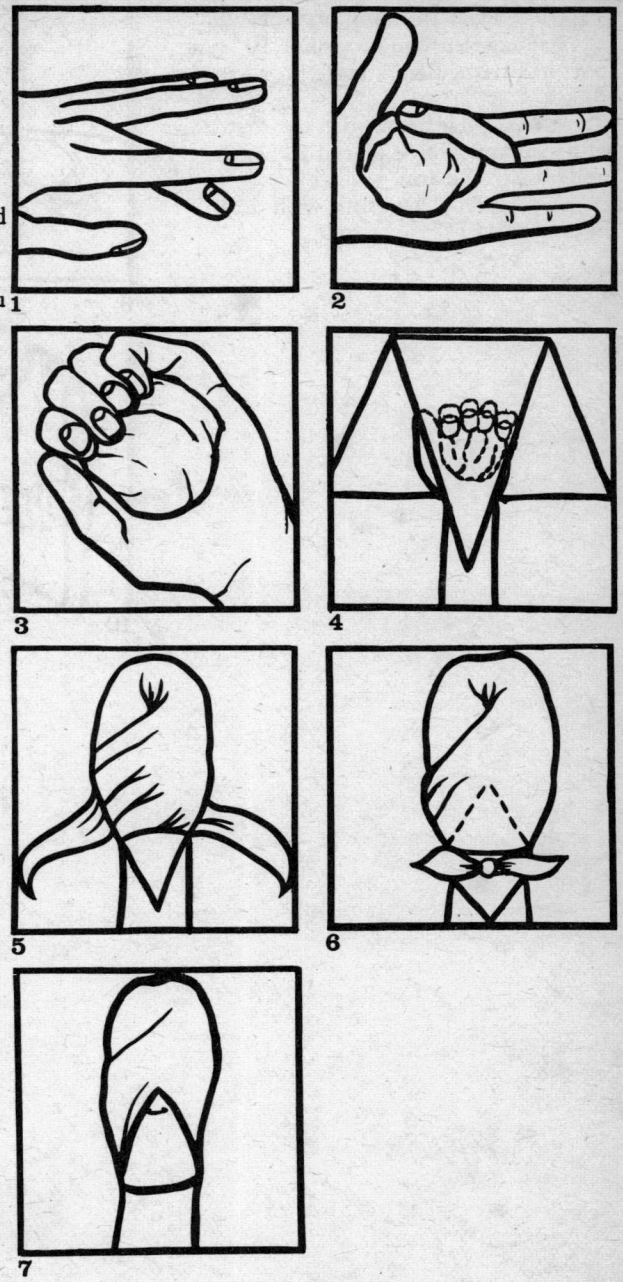

8 and 9   Place the hand on arm splint.
   Bandage the hand to splint 10   support in a triangular bandage broad arm sling.

10   A triangular bandage in the first stage of broad arm sling is placed across the chest, underneath the arm.

11   A completed arm sling with tie on injured side.

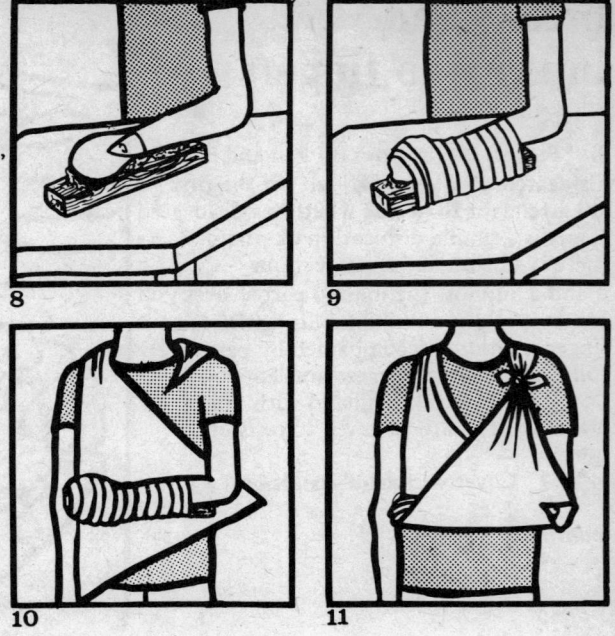

76

complicated breaks of the lower arm

1   The break of the lower arm or hand is complicated and the broken bone inside the arm has pierced the skin.
2   The wound on the skin must be cleaned with dilute antiseptic.
3   A pad to control bleeding and provide protection.
4   Bandage the wound.
5   Tie injured arm to splint.
6   Lay broad arm triangular bandage across chest.
7   Complete triangular bandage and tie it with knot over injured side.

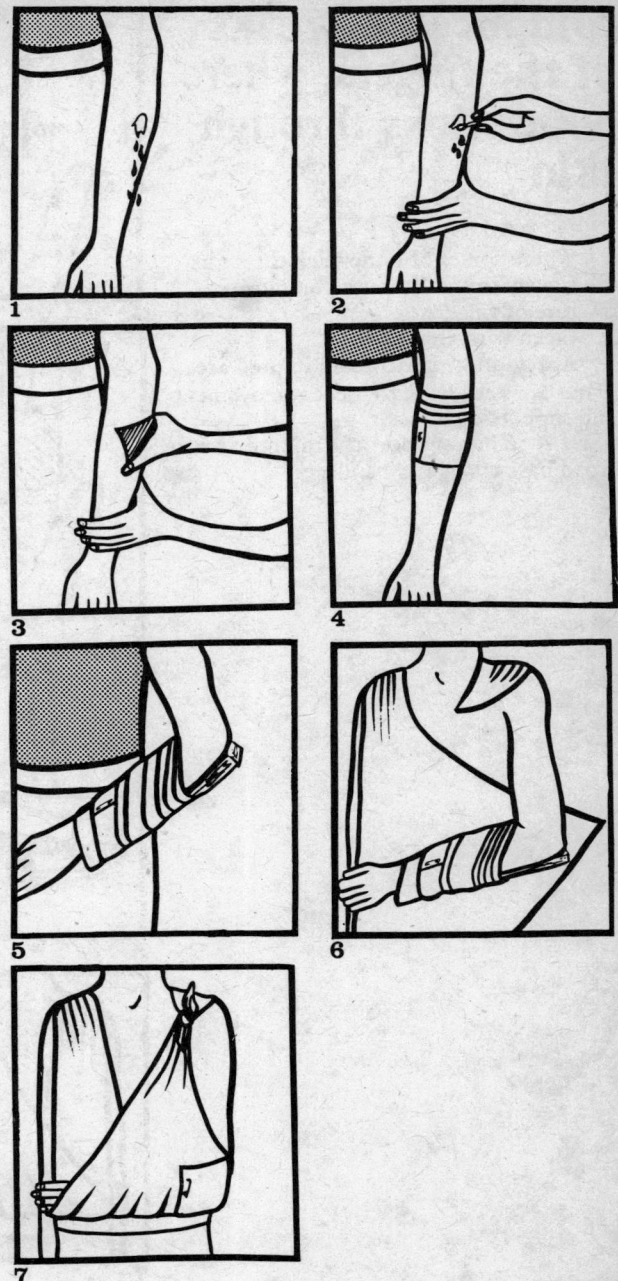

complicated breaks of the fingers, where bone sticks through skin

1 Where spikes of bone stick through the fingers this indicates a complicated fracture of fingers.

2 Clean with antiseptic.

3 Apply dressings to cover injured area.

4 and 5 Pack hand to prevent movement and support on a splint.

6 and 7 Then support the injured arm in broad base triangular bandage.

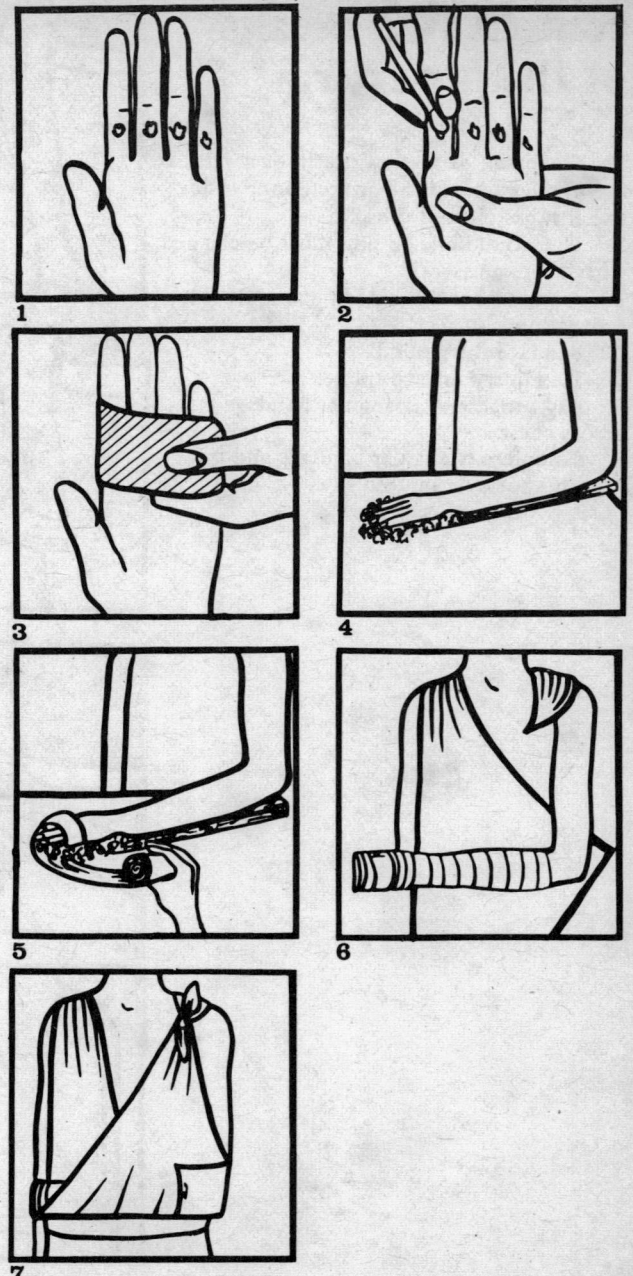

the leg
bleeding

1　Any bleeding from the *toes*, if sufficient to cause alarm, requires the leg to be elevated and direct pressure with a pad applied to the bleeding area.

2　Apply firm pressure round the ankle to reduce the blood flow to the toes.

3　Bleeding from any limb is helped in its control by elevating the limb (lifting it up in the air), calling on gravity as an additional aid in stopping the bleeding.

4　The pads that have been held on to the toes are bandaged firmly on to keep them in position.

5　Cover the whole area with a foot bandage which is made by placing the foot on a triangular bandage or triangular piece of material. The toe points to the apex point.

6　The apex point is pulled over the front of the foot.

7　The two other ends are crossed in front of the ankle, the base of the triangular bandage covering the heel.

8　Cross again at the back of the ankle and secure by tying on the front of the ankle.

9　The protruding apex of the material is turned back over and pinned to the bandage covering the top of the foot.

continued overleaf

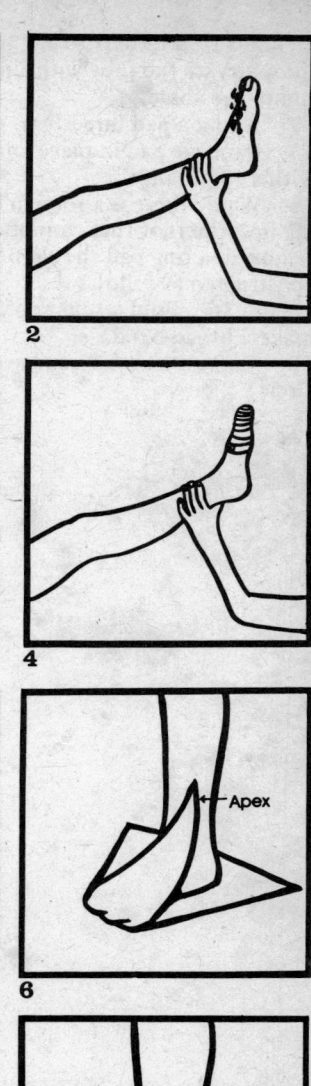

Apex

←Apex

Apex

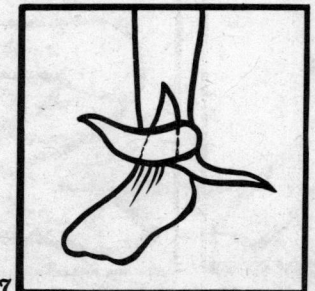

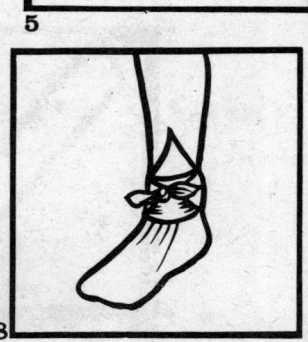

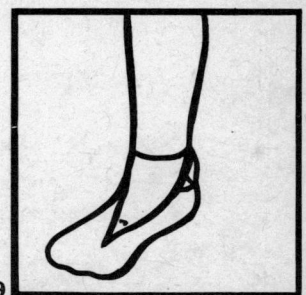

10 and 11   For *cuts to the sole of the foot*, elevate the foot with firm pressure round the ankle.

12   Apply a pad directly to the cut area.

13   Bandage pad in place and then cover with a foot bandage.

14   Where there is a foreign body sticking into the foot that cannot easily be removed, a ring pad should be constructed as follows . . .

15 and 16   Fold a square of material to make a broad bandage.

17   Twist the broad bandage into a circle.

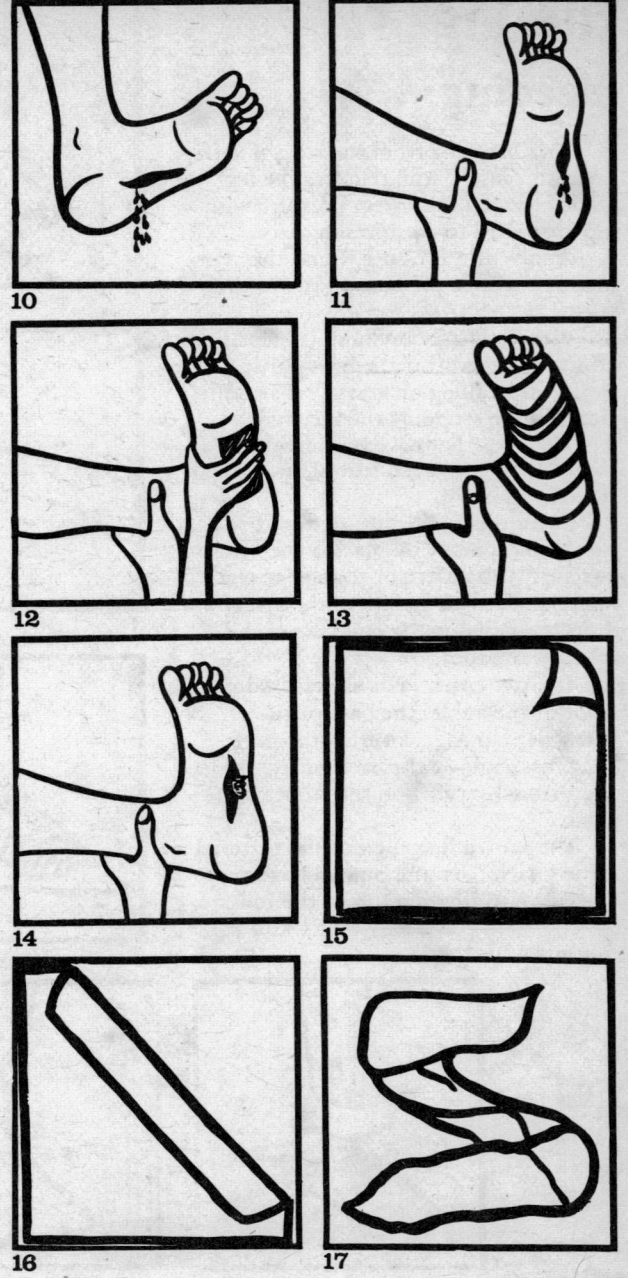

10   11

12   13

14   15

16   17

18 The ends of the bandage should be twisted round themselves to finish the ring pad.
19 The ring pad around the foreign body.
20 Apply a pad over ring and bandage.
21 Put the foot on a triangular bandage or triangular piece of material.
20 Apply a pad over ring.
21 Put the pad bandage in place, with the foot on a triangular bandage or triangular piece of material.
22 Bring the apex of triangular material over the front of the foot.
23 Cross the ends of the base of the triangular bandage round the front of the foot.
24 Bring the ends round the back and then return and tie to the front of the ankle.
25 Pin the apex point of the bandage to the top of the bandage on the foot.

continued overleaf

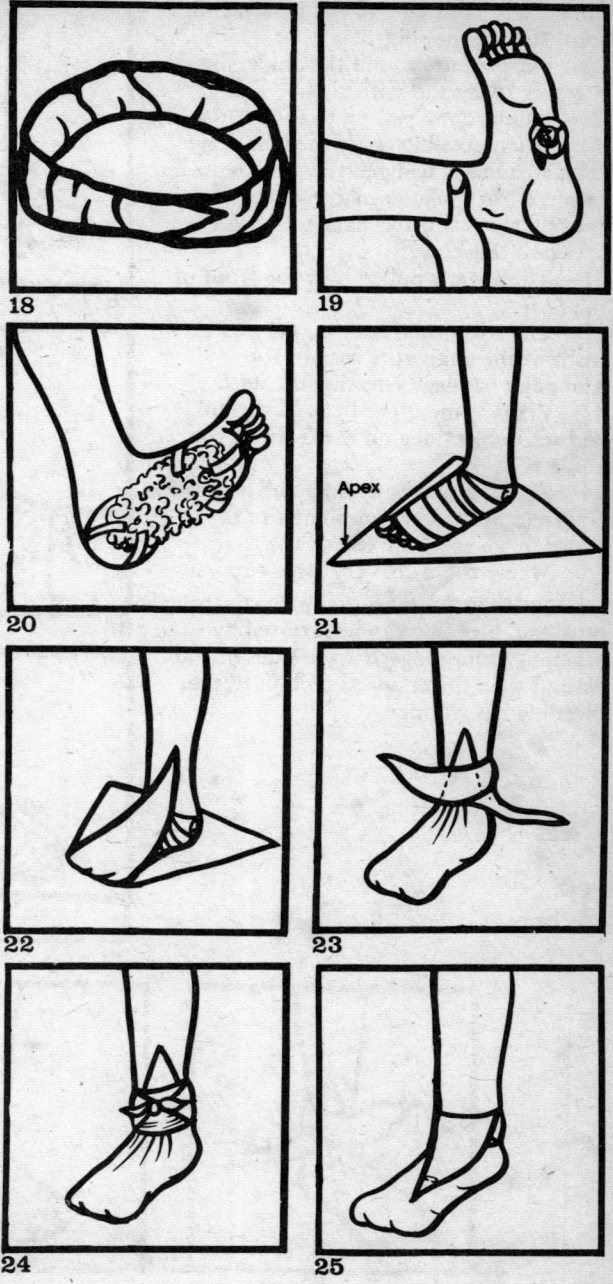

18 19 20 21 22 23 24 25

26 and 27   For cuts to the front of the foot, elevate the foot . . .

28   Put pressure round the ankle, direct pressure to wound with a pad.

29   Bandage the pad on to the foot.

30   When possible cover the whole area with a bandage, using a triangular bandage or piece of triangular material. Put the foot on the triangular bandage with the toes pointing towards the apex.

31   The apex is pulled over the front of the foot.

32   The two other ends are crossed in front of the ankle, the base of the triangular bandage covering the heel.

33   Cross again at the back of the ankle and secure by tying on the front of the ankle.

34   The protruding apex of the material is turned back over and pinned to the bandage covering the top of the foot.

Where there are very large cuts on the foot that cannot initially be controlled by a pad, bleeding can be arrested by pinching firmly together the sides of the wound with finger and thumb until the bleeding has stopped.

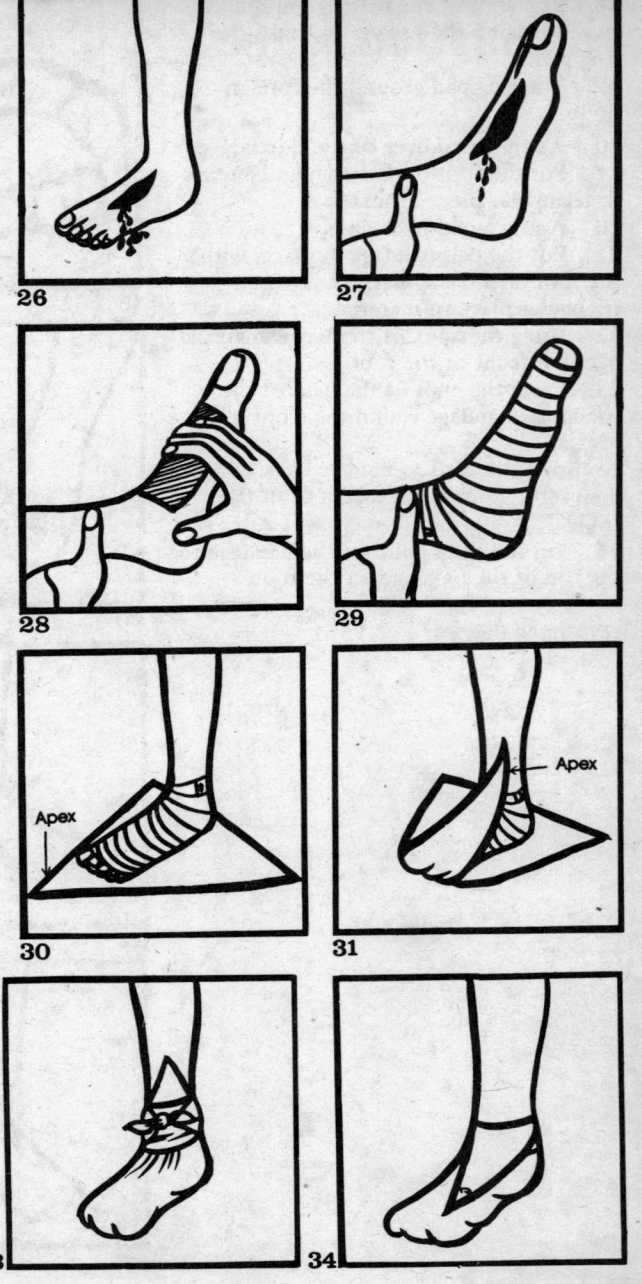

amputation of toes

1 to 3   In an accident where the toes have been amputated, if one or more toes are amputated, then the best way of reducing the blood flow is, initially, putting a tourniquet round the ankle. A tourniquet is made by tying a stout bandage or thick material round the ankle in a loop. A stick is put through the top of the loop and then rotated in a clockwise direction until the pressure is such that no blood comes through.

4   When the tourniquet has controlled the bleeding, a firm pad should be bandaged on to the bleeding areas.

5 and 6   The pad is held in position by firm bandaging to and fro across the stumps, starting and finishing well below the amputation site. This is then anchored by firm bandaging *around* the foot.

7. The tourniquet should be released to see if the bandage and padding has controlled the bleeding. The foot should always be elevated in any severe bleeding from it to reduce the blood flow. Where the pad and bandage are not containing the bleeding, the tourniquet should be re-applied and released for 1 minute every 20 minutes to see whether bleeding has been controlled, until expert medical help has arrived.

The bandaged foot with amputated toes can be kept in the best position, when possible, by applying a foot bandage, details for which can be found on the preceding page.

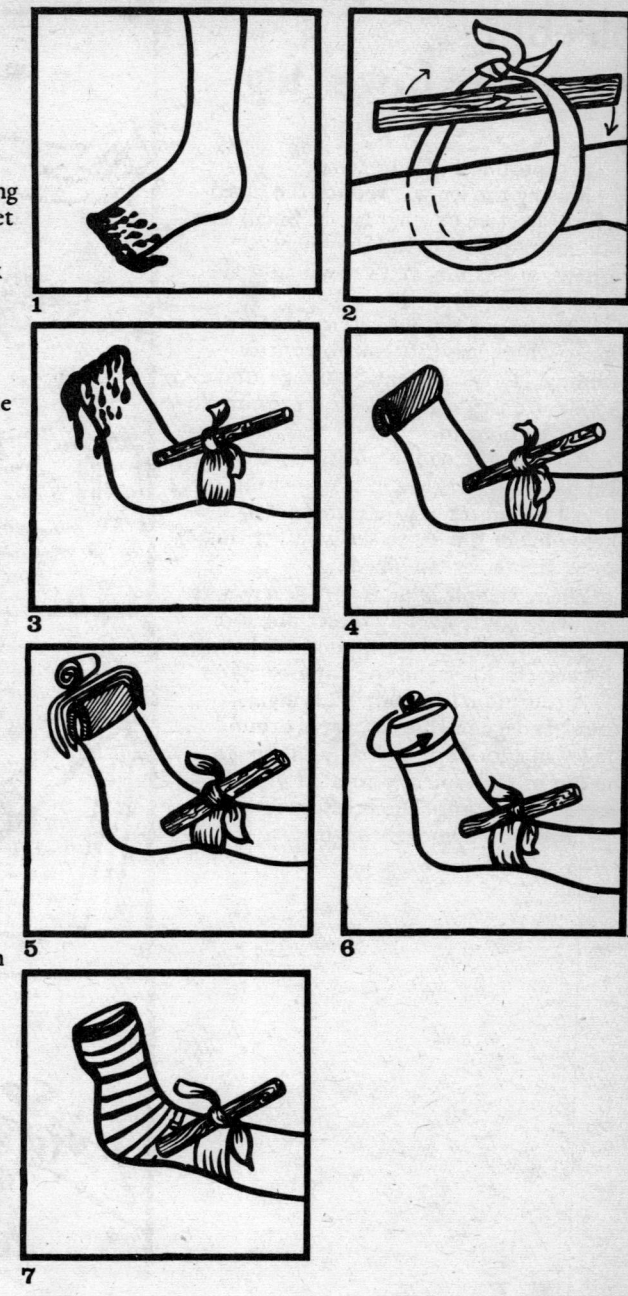

bleeding
from the lower leg

1   A typical lower leg wound.
2   Raising the leg will reduce the bleeding, irrespective of what types. Small cuts may not require this; all they need, perhaps, is cleaning and a small adhesive dressing being applied.
3   For the patient with a large cut on the leg where it is difficult to control bleeding, lay the patient on the ground and elevate the leg, apply firm pressure to the cut with a pad.
4   Bandage the pad in position with firm bandaging. Leave in this position for 10 to 15 minutes before transporting. Slowly lower the leg to see whether this causes an increase in bleeding.
5   Where the bleeding is very severe and cannot be controlled by direct pressure, a tourniquet should be applied to the leg between the knee and the cut area.
6   A tourniquet is made by tying a stout bandage or thick material around the leg in a loop. A stick is put through the top of the loop and rotated in a clockwise direction until the pressure is such that no blood comes through.

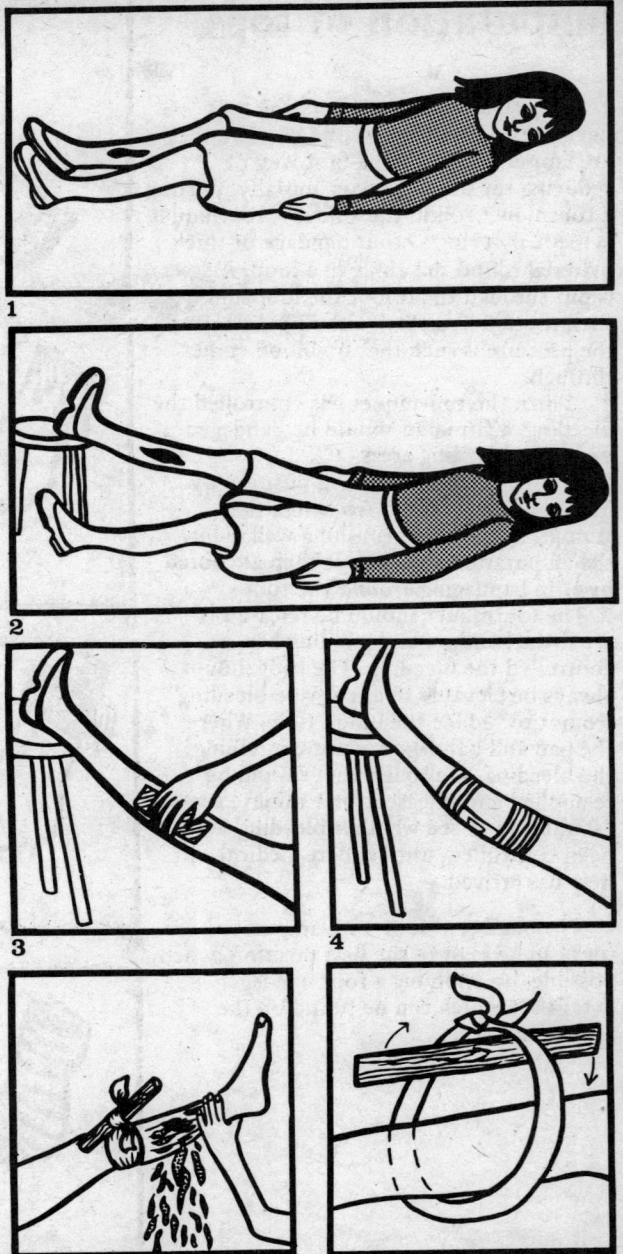

7   Apply a dressing to area, with tourniquet still in position.
8   Bandage leg firmly, keeping leg elevated.
9   With leg still elevated, remove tourniquet to see if bleeding has been controlled.

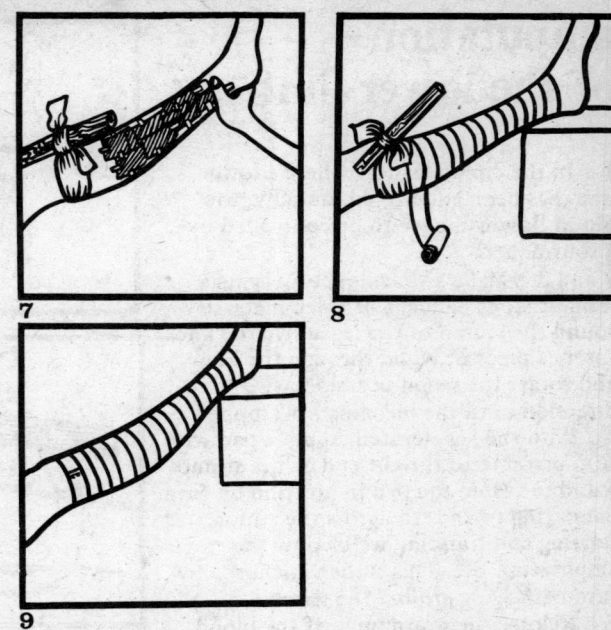

bleeding from a varicose vein

1   When a varicose vein has been cut, the bleeding is often excessive, and it should be treated as a severe cut to the leg. The patient should be laid on the ground and the affected leg lifted 2 ft. off the ground and kept in this position. Apply a pad to bleeding area.
2   If the cut is extensive, pressure should be applied above and below the varicose vein, as well as directly on it, as bleeding from varicose veins, as opposed to arterial bleeding, can bleed from both ends of the cut. Two firmly tied bandages — as opposed to tourniquets — should control varicose bleeding.
3   With limb elevated, bandage pad in place.

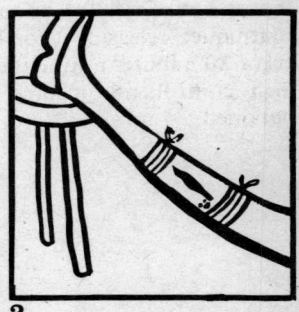

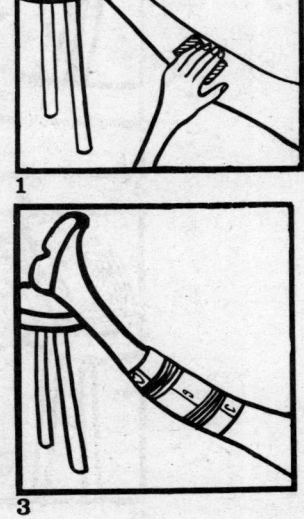

amputation of the lower limb

1 In the circumstances where a lower limb has been amputated, initially, the blood flow will have to be controlled by a tourniquet.

2 and 3 Make a tourniquet by tying a loop of stout bandage or thick material round the stump of the leg above the knee. Insert a piece of wood through the loop and rotate the wood in a clockwise direction until the bleeding has stopped.

4 With the leg elevated, apply a pad with firm pressure to the cut end of the stump.

5 and 6 Hold the pad in position by firm bandaging to and fro across the stump, starting and finishing well below the amputation site. This is then anchored by firm bandaging *around* the stump.

7 Release the tourniquet. If the blood flow is not controlled, re-apply the tourniquet, releasing it for 1 minute every 20 minutes until either the bleeding is controlled or medical help has been obtained.

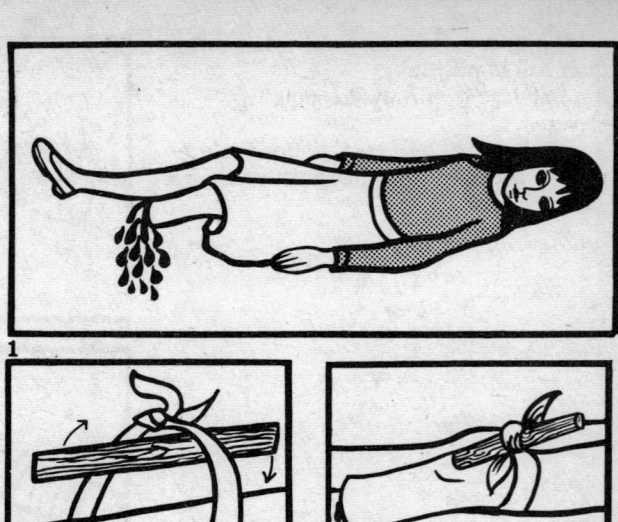

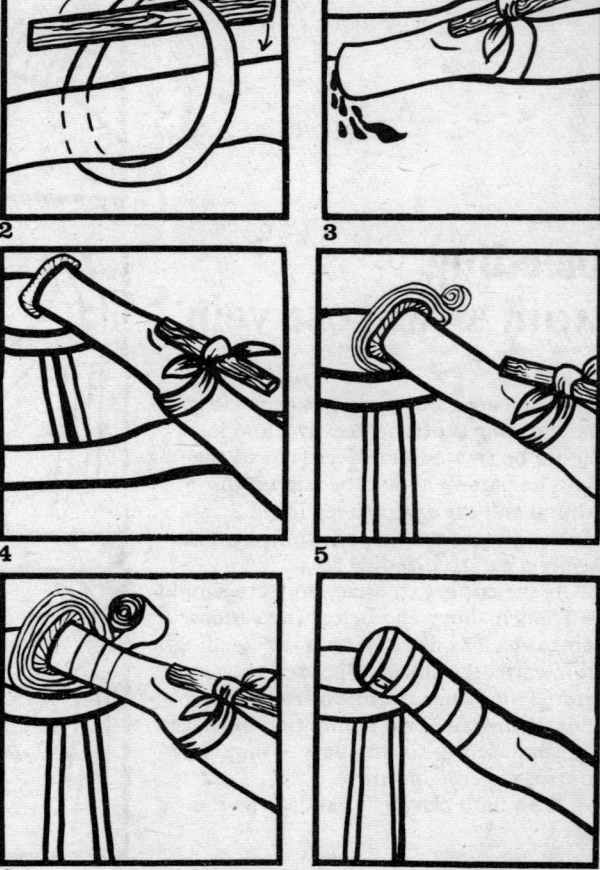

cuts to the knee

1 Cuts to the knee should be treated under the same principles as any other cut on the leg. The limb should be elevated if the bleeding is severe, and direct pressure should be applied with a pad to the cut area to reduce the bleeding. The one difficulty with injuries to the knee is keeping a bandage in place. Having put on a firm dressing, the whole dressing can be kept in place by a knee bandage made out of a triangular bandage or a triangular piece of material. Place the apex of the triangle on the thigh with the base of the triangle just below the knee.
2 Pick up the lower two ends and cross them first behind the calf, and then again up to meet on top of the thigh, and tie to top of the thigh.
3 Bring the protruding apex down to pin on the body of the bandage.

bleeding from the thigh

1 Bleeding from the thigh.
2 This can be controlled by elevating the limb and applying a pressure pad, i.e. pressing a firm pad of clean or sterile material on to the bleeding area itself.
3 Fix the pad in place by bandaging. When the bleeding is controlled and the bandage secured, the limb can be lowered.

continued overleaf

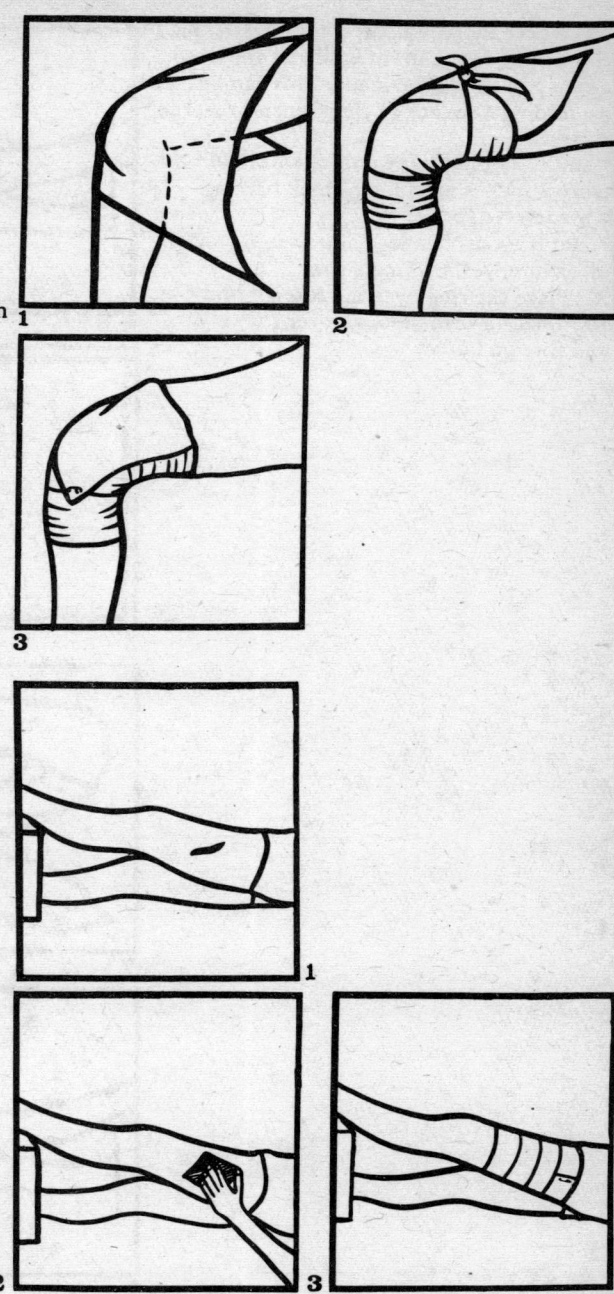

87

4 Where there is a foreign body sticking in the wound that cannot easily be removed, a ring pad should be made. This can be made by folding a square of clean linen or sterile material.

5 and 6 Fold in one corner and then fold every 2 inches until long, thick bandage is made.

7 and 8 Curl bandage and then tie ends on themselves, making a ring.

9 Place the ring over the foreign body.

10 Place a firm dressing over the ring and foreign body.

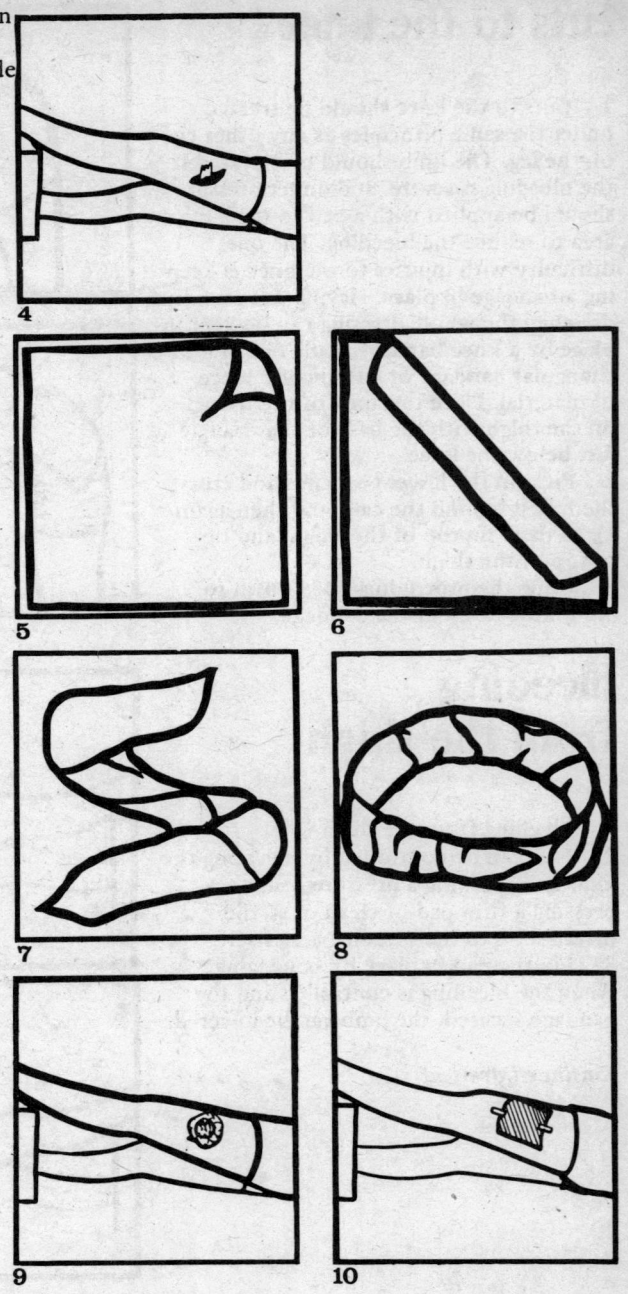

11 Bandage to maintain in position.
12 Where the laceration is long and cannot initially be controlled by a pad, bleeding can be reduced by pinching the sides of the wound together.

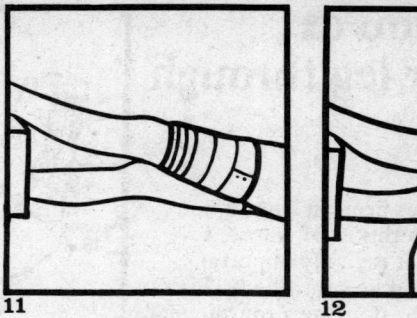

13 One of the difficulties in keeping bandages on the thigh and buttocks is that they will slip down. For burns, minor cuts and abrasions to the buttocks and upper thigh, a hip bandage will cover the underlying skin. Tie a bandage round the waist.
14 Then tuck the apex of the triangular bandage underneath.
15 Tie the ends at the base of the triangle then cross behind the inside of the thigh.
16 Bring round to the outside and tie, and bring the apex of the triangle back over the knot and pin to the substance of the cloth.

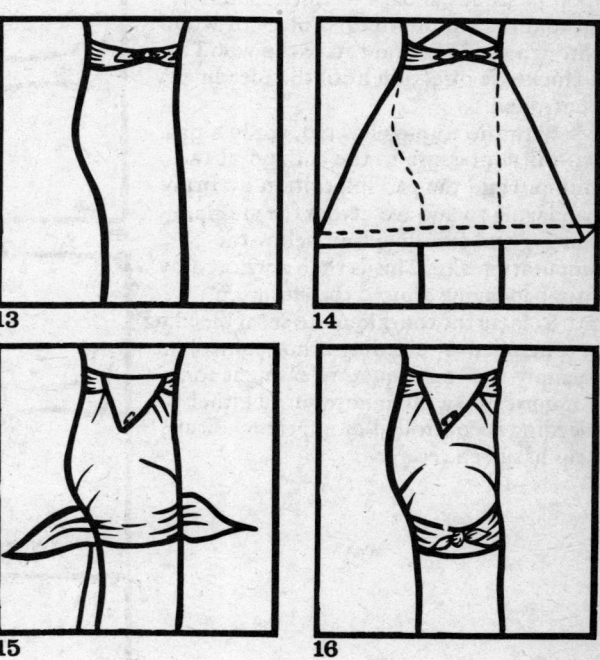

amputation of the upper leg through the thigh

1 Where there has been an amputation from the upper leg this is, of course, a severe injury, and it is vitally important that bleeding should be controlled. This can perhaps only be done by a tourniquet in the initial stages

2 and 3 Make a tourniquet by tying a loop of stout bandage or thick material around the stump. Insert a piece of wood through the loop and rotate the wood in a clockwise direction until the bleeding is controlled.

4 With the stump elevated, apply a pad with firm pressure to the cut end of the stump. Hold the pad in position by firm bandaging to and fro across the stump, starting and finishing well below the amputation site. This is then anchored by firm bandaging *around* the stump.

5 Release the tourniquet to see if bleeding is controlled. If bleeding is not controlled, re-apply the tourniquet, releasing it for 1 minute every 20 minutes until either the bleeding is controlled or expert medical help has been received.

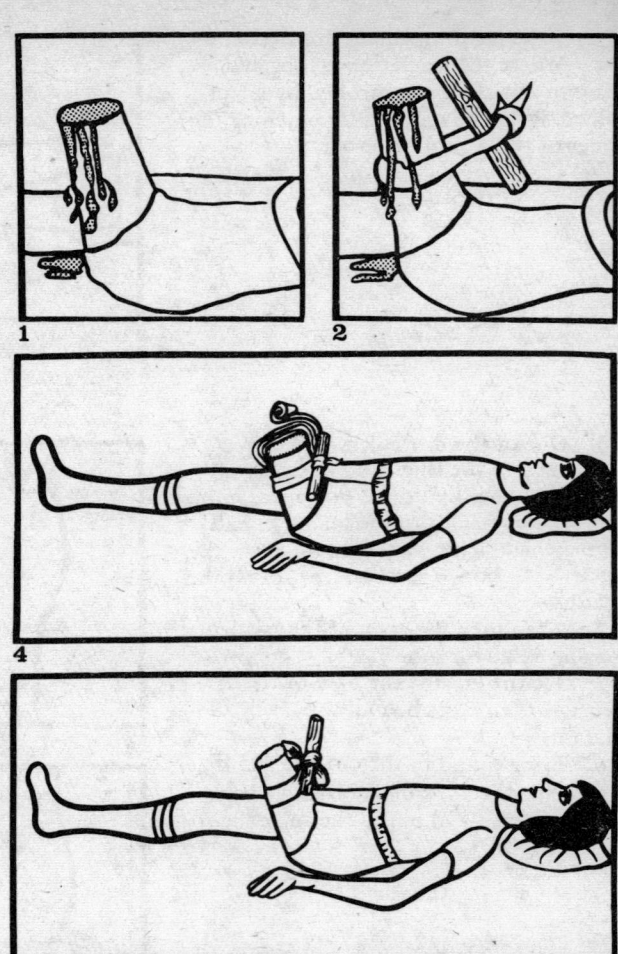

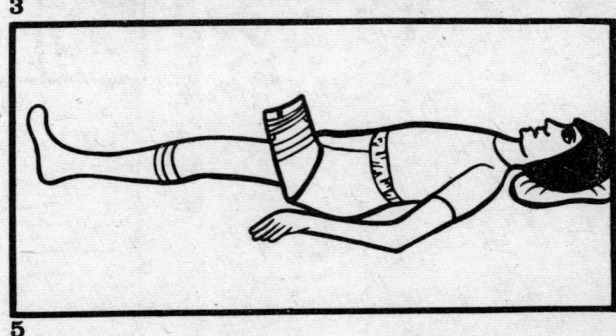

burns and scalds of the leg

The general principles for the treatment of all burns are:
- Take away from the heat.
- Take the heat away from the burn.
- Protect from contamination and infection.

1   A burnt foot, with blisters.
2   The initial treatment is to pour cold water over the burn or scalded area. Do not prick blisters — they provide a sterile covering to the burnt area.
3   When possible put on paraffin gauze dressings as these protect sticking to both skin and bandage.
4   Cover with either sterile or clean linen or bandage.
5   A severe burn to the foot in which a sock is involved
6   Treat by pouring cold water over burnt area.
7   Do not try to pick off material that is embedded in the burns, but cut through the material so there is no constricting bend round the foot.
8   Encase the whole foot in sterile or clean linen — a pillow case will very often do in these circumstances and will provide protection whilst the severe burn is taken to a medical centre for specialist treatment.

continued overleaf

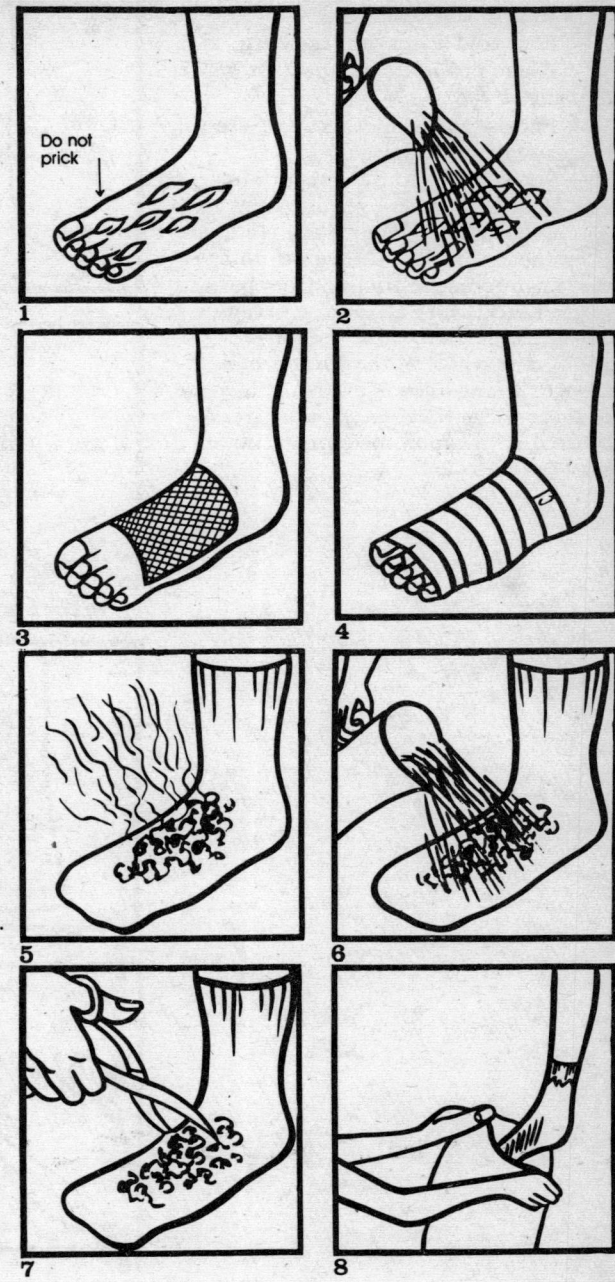

9   Burns to the lower leg.

10   Pour cold water over the burn.

11   Where possible apply paraffin gauze dressings.

12   Enclose the whole area, plus dressing, in clean linen or bandage.

13   Severe burns to the upper or lower leg.

14   Pour cold water over the burnt area.

15   Do not try to remove any clothing from the leg, but cut through clothing that might cause restriction from burn to thigh. Keep the leg elevated as severe burning is likely to cause swelling.

16   Cover whole of the burnt area with clean or sterile linen — often a pillowcase or sheet will suffice. Keep burnt area covered until expert medical attention has been obtained.

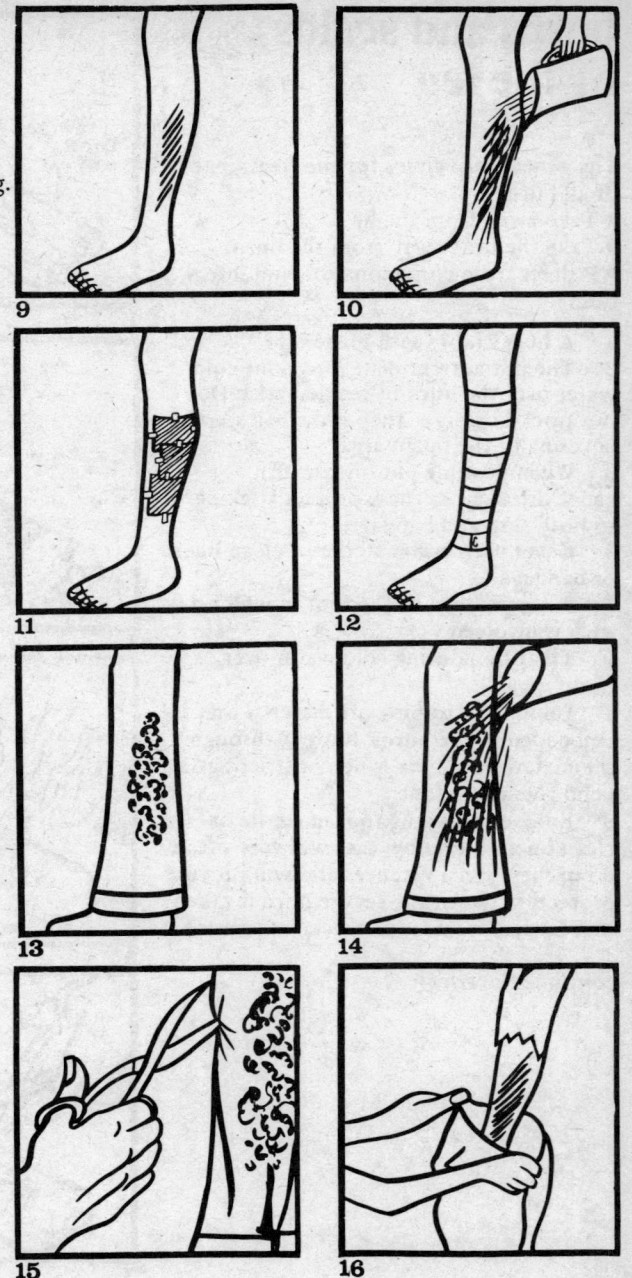

breaks
and dislocations
of the leg

A break or dislocation is suspected when
there is pain and deformity in the limb.
It is extremely difficult for a first aid
attendant to differentiate between a dislocation and a break, and most often an x-ray
will be required; so, as a general principle,
all pain and deformity in bones should be
considered and treated as a break until
proved otherwise.

breaks
and dislocations
of the toes

1   Suspect the toes are broken or dislocated if they are out of position and
causing pain.
2   Reduce the pain by immobilising, by
packing round with soft padding, using any
soft material that is available.
3   Keep the soft tissue in place by an
enclosing bandage round the foot.

continued overleaf

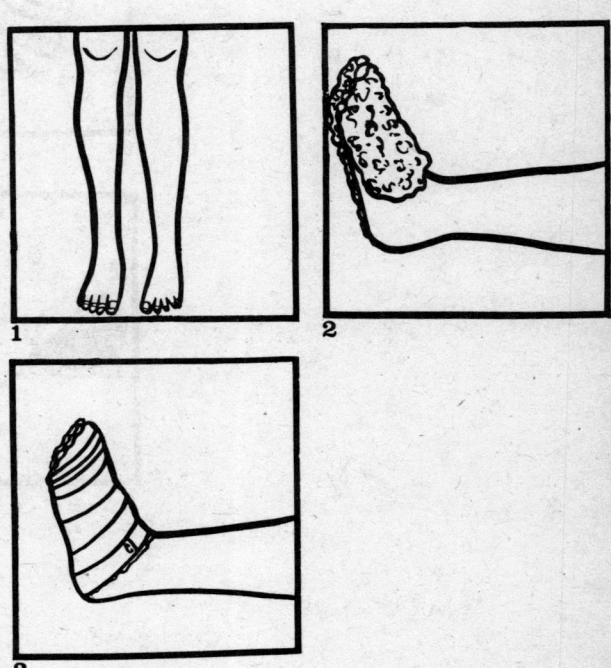

4 to 6   Where the injury is minimal this will be sufficient, but where there is considerable trauma and bony damage, the foot should be supported, ideally with an L-shaped splint, the padded foot being rested upon it and fixed to it with a bandage. This type of splint is most useful for any break of the foot or the lower ankle, keeping the foot still for transporting the patient to hospital or for expert medical help.

7   For any broken bone of the leg, the splinting of the injured leg is done by tying to the uninjured leg, and is always part — sometimes all — of the treatment required.

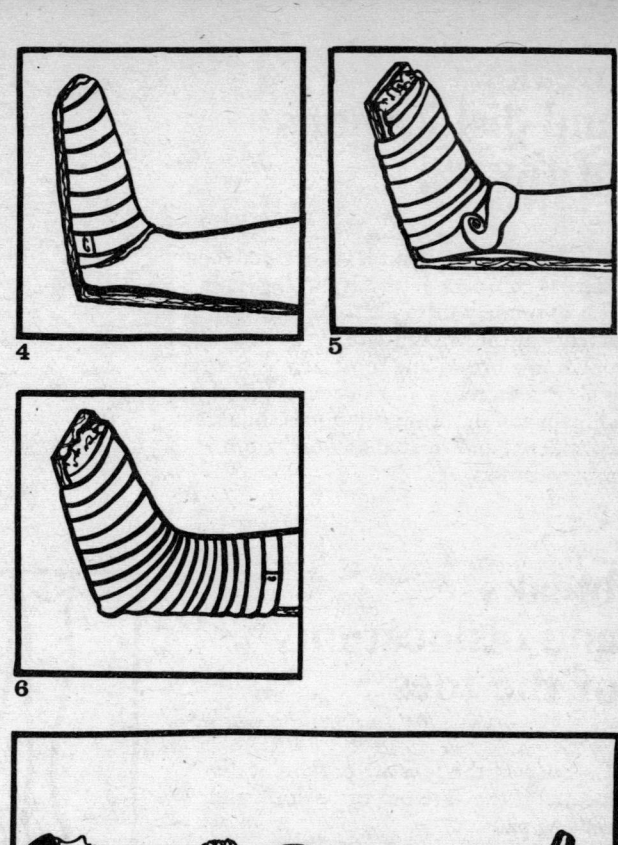

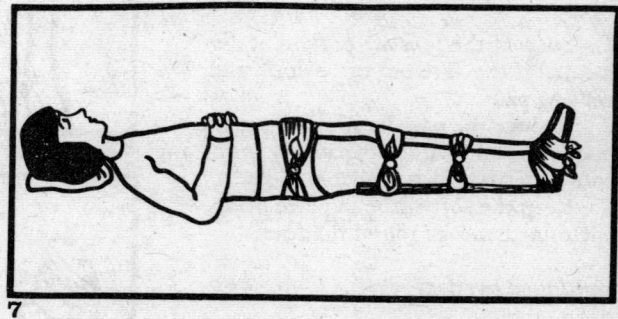

8 to 11   Where the break of the toe is not
a simple one, and bone has penetrated the
skin making it complicated, a dressing
should be first applied to the individual
toe before padding and bandaging.

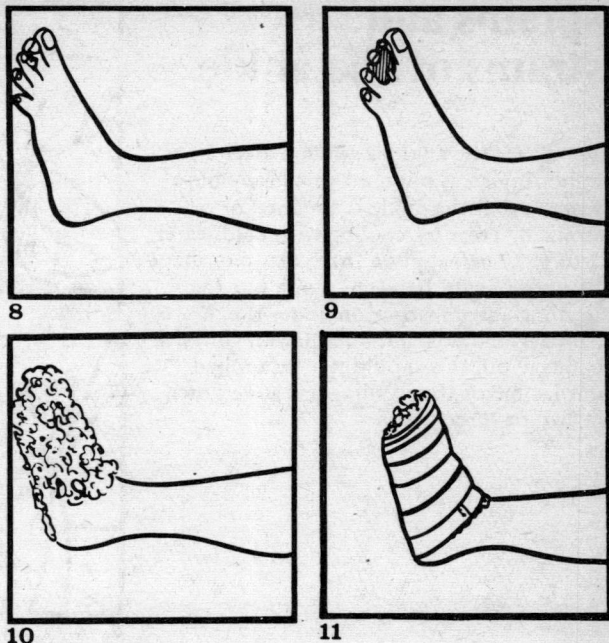

12   An injury that is not uncommon
round the ankle is a rupture or break of
the Achilles tendon, the ligament that is
attached to the back of the heel. Suspect
that the Achilles tendon is broken if there
is pain in the ankle and a lump just above
the ankle with a depression at the back
of the heel which is not present on the
other side.
13   Immobilise by bandaging and keeping
the patient's weight off his foot.

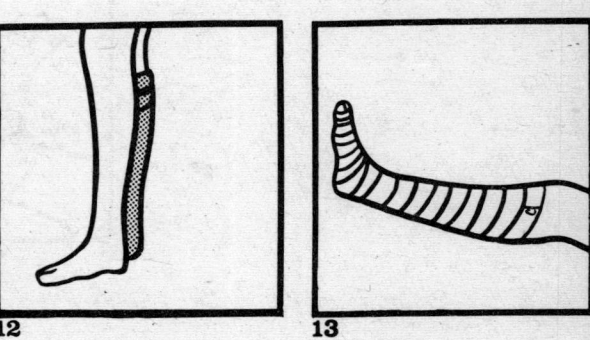

sprains and strains of the ankle

1   Where the ankle is swollen after a minor injury as opposed to a heavy blow, suspect that the ankle is sprained or strained. Treat by cooling with cold water.
2 to 5   Then apply a firm cotton or crepe 'figure-of-eight' bandage. Look out for swelling and constriction under the bandage. Do not, initially, put an adhesive bandage on; this should not be applied until some of the swelling has gone down in two or three days.

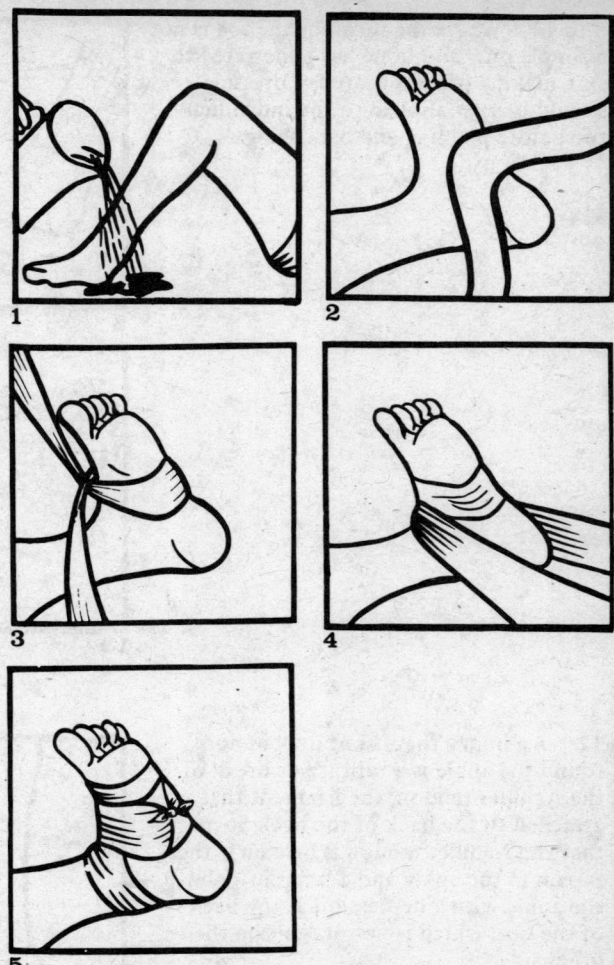

breaks of the ankle

1   Suspect that the ankle or lower leg is broken if there is pain and deformity round the ankle and the injury to the ankle has been more than that which would be likely to cause a sprain. Treat by immobilising to lessen the pain and stop broken ends doing tissue damage inside the limb.

2   Cut through any restrictive clothing that might be round the foot or lower leg.

3   Bandage the lower leg to a splint with a figure-of-eight bandage holding the ankle to the splint.

4   Tie the bad leg to the good leg to avoid jarring in transport.

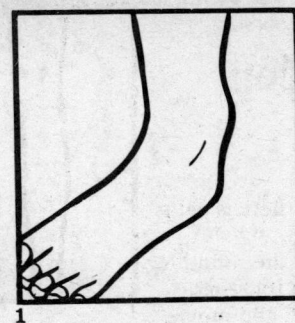

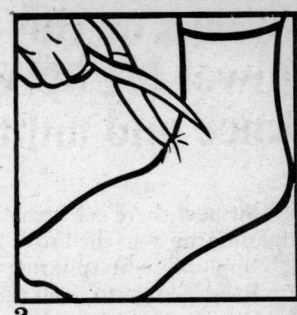

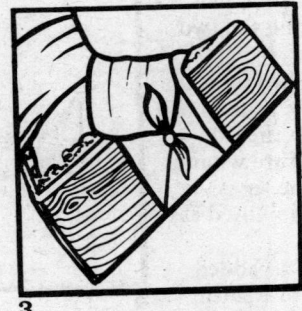

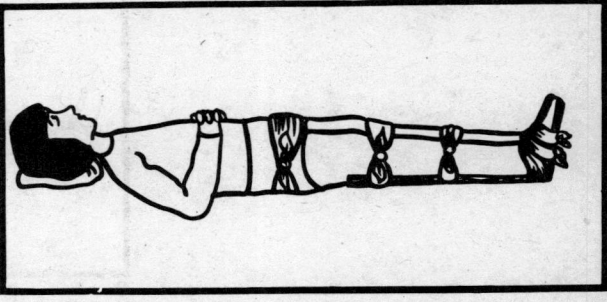

breaks of the lower leg between knee and ankle

1 Suspect there is a break if there is pain and deformity in the lower leg.

2 Immobilise by splinting to the sound leg.

3 Bandage feet to keep them together.

4 During transportation, pain and movement are decreased if a splint is applied to the whole leg before splinting the two legs together.

5 Sometimes there are complications in breaks to the lower leg and the broken end of the bone protrudes through the skin.

6 In this case, the skin puncture wound must first be dressed before the leg is immobilised, then the leg immobilised as for a simple break.

7 The leg is then splinted to a padded splint going the whole length of the leg.

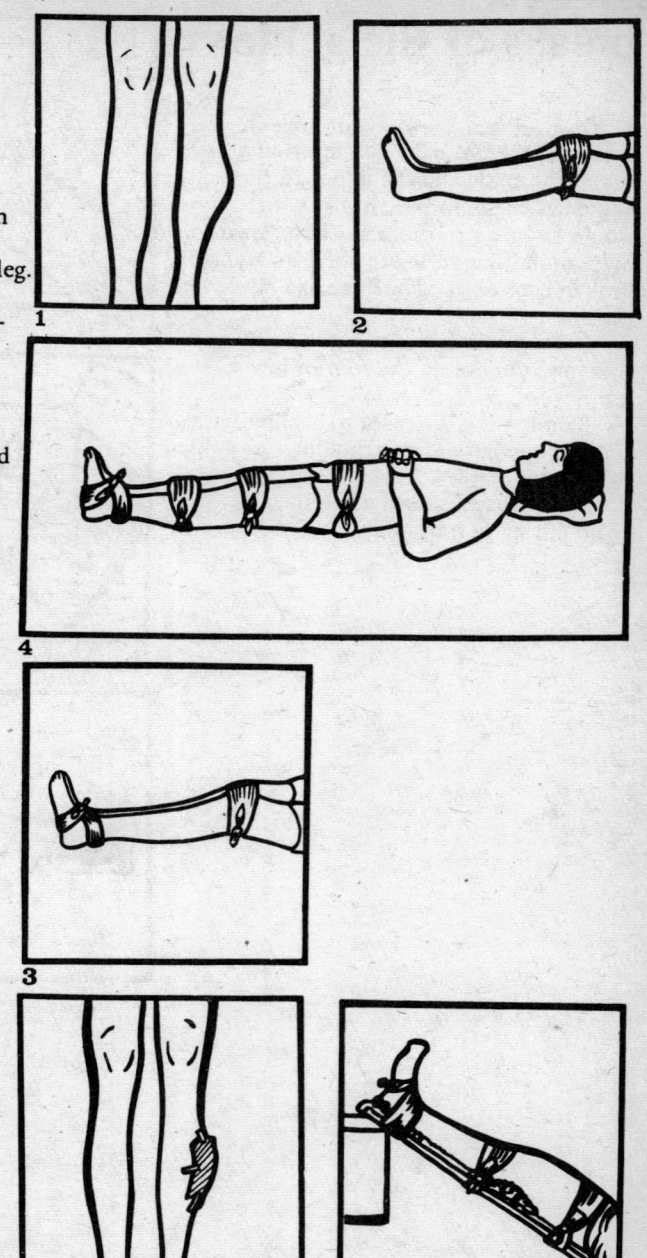

broken knee-cap

1   Suspect that the knee-cap is broken if, following a blow or severe strain, there is pain and swelling of the knee joint, tenderness in front of the knee and, in some cases, a depression in the knee-cap of the affected side as opposed to the un-affected side.
2   Treat by elevating the leg . . .
3   . . . then place leg on a padded splint. Tie round the ankle, mid-calf and mid-thigh, to prevent movement.
4   If the patient is to be transported, tying both legs together will further reduce pain and discomfort.

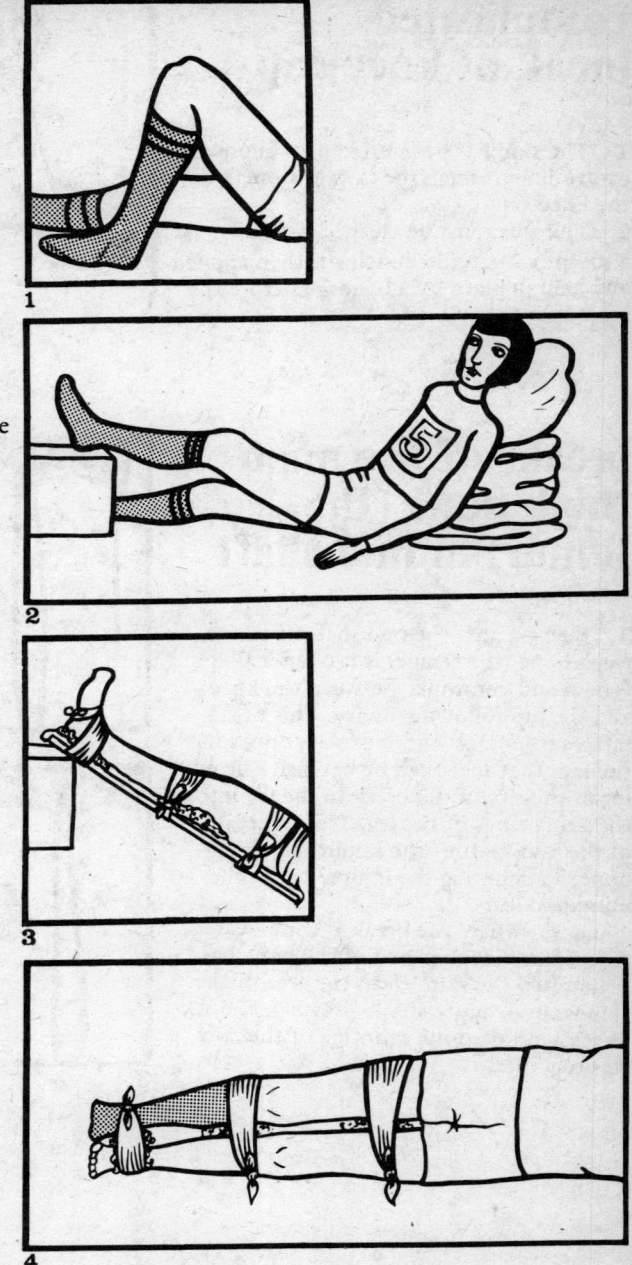

complicated break of knee-cap

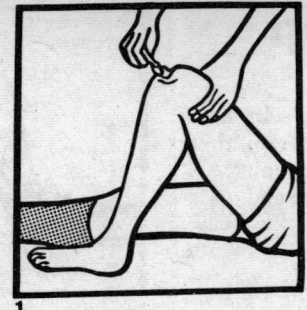
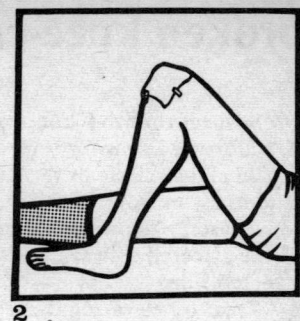

1   The skin has been broken and bone is protruding through the skin in a break of the knee-cap.

2   The area must be cleaned with an antiseptic. A sterile dressing is then applied and held in place by a bandage before the leg is splinted.

breaks of the main thigh bone (the femur) in mid-shaft

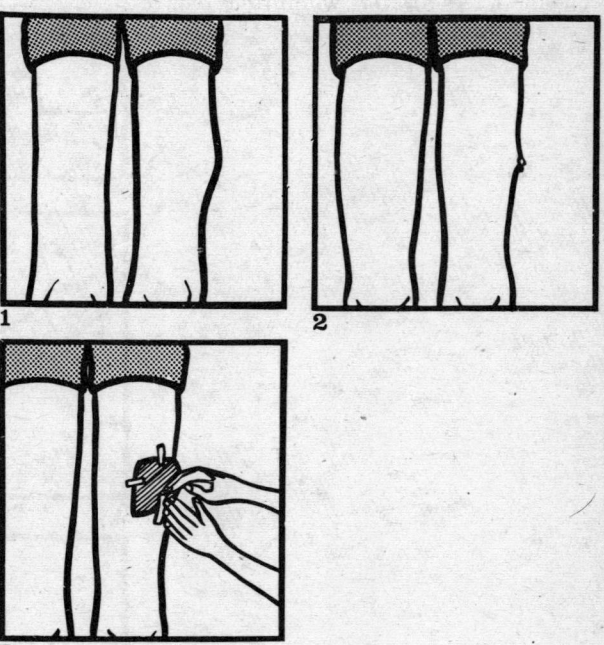

1   Suspect that the mid shaft of the thigh bone (the femur) is broken if there is pain and deformity between the knee and the hip following injury. This break differs from most other broken bones in the fact that there can be extensive bleeding at the site of the break in the leg into the soft tissues of the leg. Treat a break of the mid-shaft of the femur, i.e. thigh bone, by splinting the injured leg to the uninjured leg.

2 and 3   Where the break is complicated, that is if the broken end of the bone has penetrated the skin, clean the area of the skin wound, apply sterile dressing, and fix in place prior to the splinting of the two legs together.

4 As well as the first aid procedures for splinting the leg it is important to keep an eye on the general condition of the patient to see whether he is showing signs of blood loss, i.e. faintness, rapidly increasing pulse, volume of the pulse decreasing.

5 The legs are splinted together by first placing a padding between the two legs then, with a series of ties, tying the feet together, the mid calf above and below the knee and mid thigh, thus immobilising the legs.

6 When possible further immobilisation can be achieved by placing a wooden splint from the arm-pit to the foot of the injured side and including it in the tying bandages splinting together the two legs. Further ties will also be required at the top of the splint, half-way up the chest and round the hips.

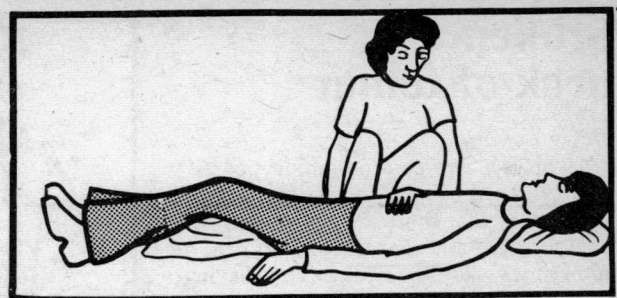

4

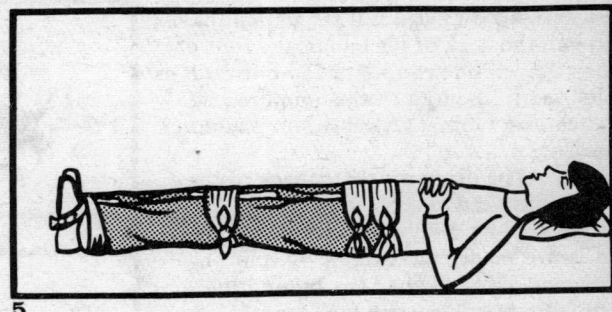

5

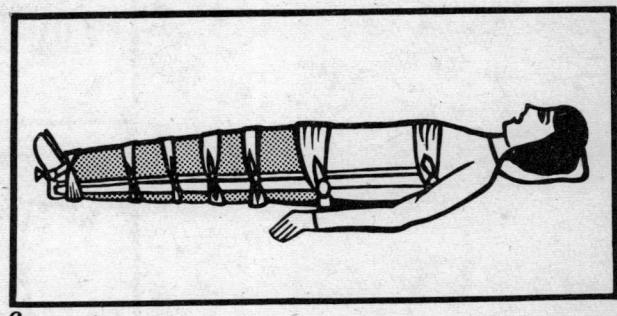

6

broken
neck of femur

1   This is a very common injury, particularly in old people, and is complicated
by the fact that there are not always
obvious signs and that the patient can
sometimes walk, the broken ends having
compacted. This is a break that can very
easily be missed.

2   A significant sign is if the patient has
broken the neck of his femur, the foot of
the affected side turns laterally outwards as
opposed to the foot of the uninjured side
which, in a normal rest position, is almost
upright.

3 to 5   The diagnosis that a neck of the
femur has been broken can only be
established by x-ray investigations. The
patient is made comfortable by splinting
the good leg to the bad leg, by multiple
ties from feet, knee and hip areas.

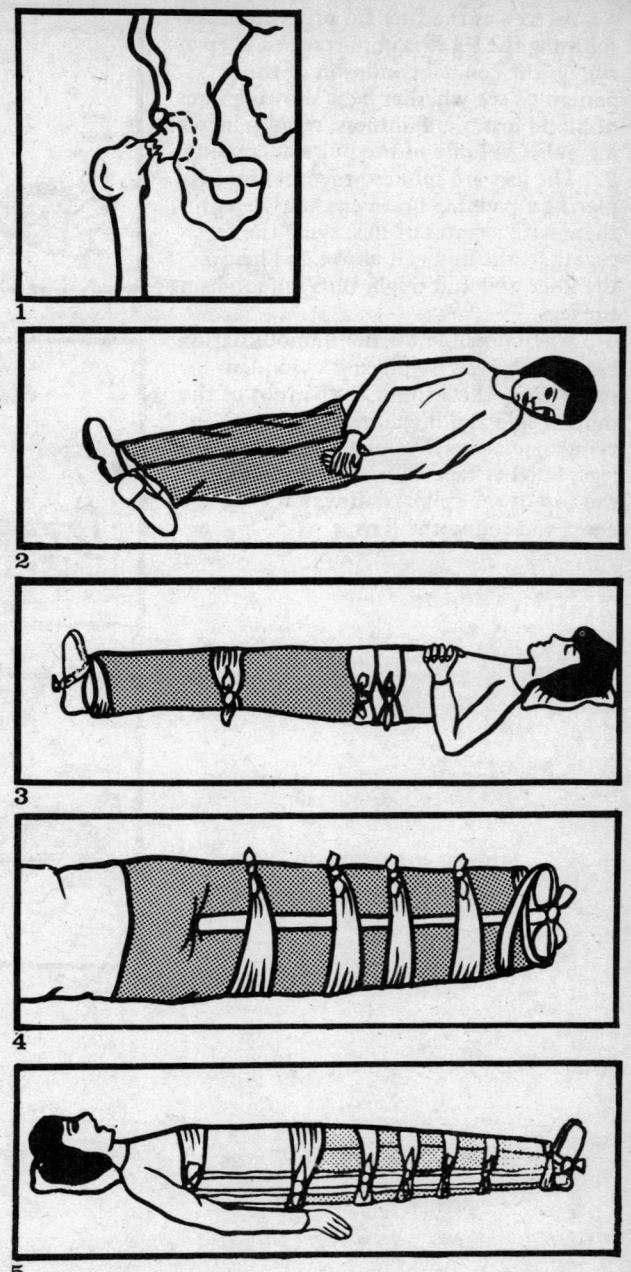

the chest

bleeding from the chest

1   Superficial bleeding from small cuts in the chest.
2   Control the bleeding by applying a pad of clean linen or sterile material, applying direct pressure over the bleeding area. Unless the patient has some other limiting injury, he is better sitting or being supported in a sitting position.
3   Pad being held in position by firm bandaging.
4   Where the chest wound is not severe, and in either burns or multiple superficial cuts, the chest needs to be covered. This can be done with a triangular bandage or triangular piece of material. Just lie a triangular bandage over the chest with the apex of the bandage going over one shoulder.
5   Tie the two ends of the base of the triangle round the back.
6   Join the apex of the triangle to the knot of the knotted two ends with a short bandage.
7   Secure the bandage in position.

continued overleaf

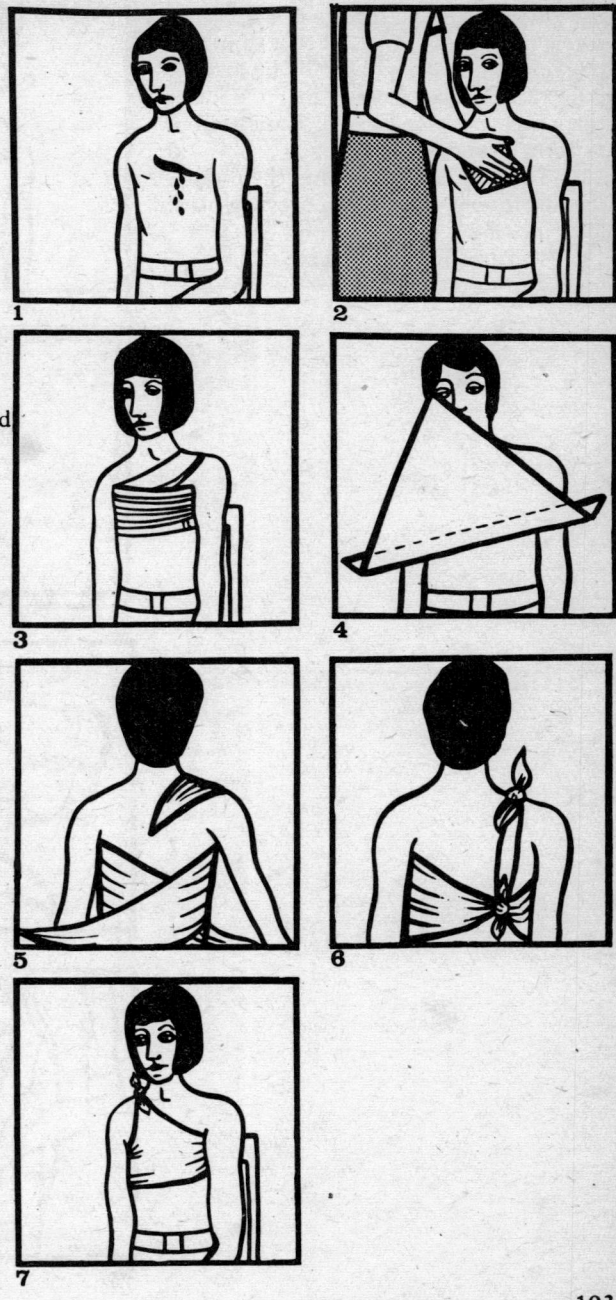

103

8   Where there is a foreign body, or foreign bodies, in a wound that cannot be removed, a ring pad should be made.

9 to 12   Fold a square of material into a thick bandage then twisting it on itself to form a ring.

13   The ring is placed round the protruding foreign body and a dressing placed over the ring.

14   The dressing and ring are firmly bandaged to the chest.

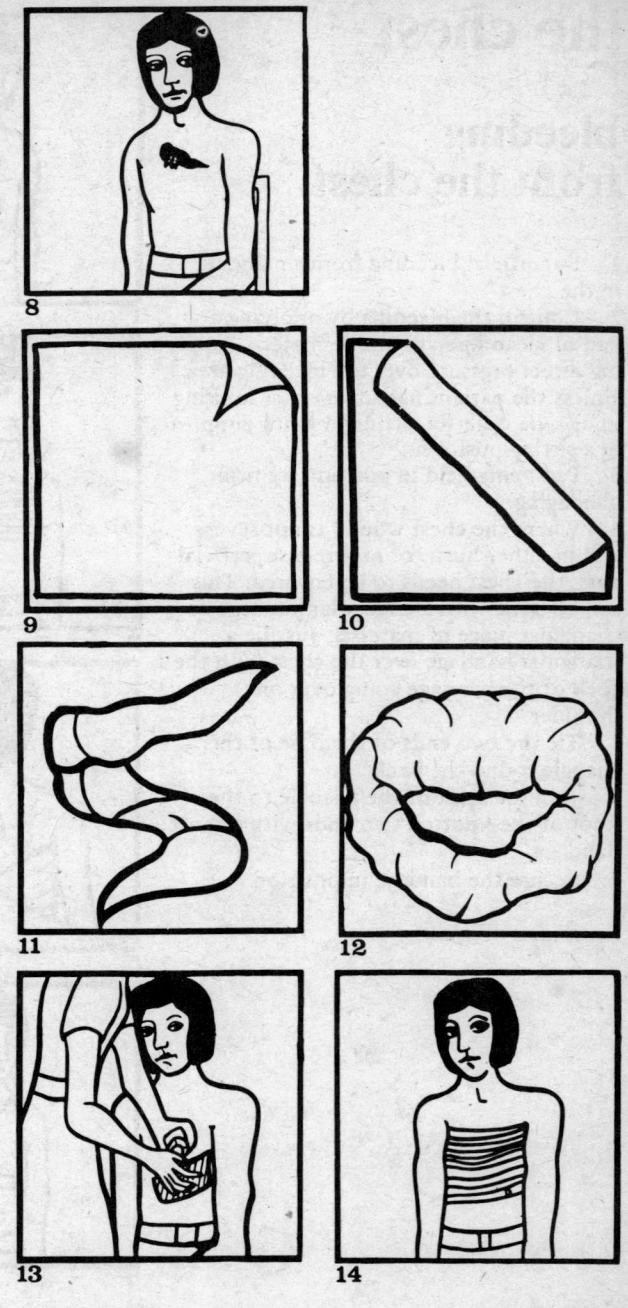

8

9

10

11

12

13

14

15   For superficial wounds or burns to the
back of the chest, where it is needed to cover
and protect the chest, a similar bandage to
the chest bandage can be used.

16   In this case a triangular bandage is
laid over the back of the chest with the
apex going over one shoulder.

17   The ends of the base are brought
round to the front of the chest and tied.
Then the apex and tie of the base ends
are joined together by a short bandage.

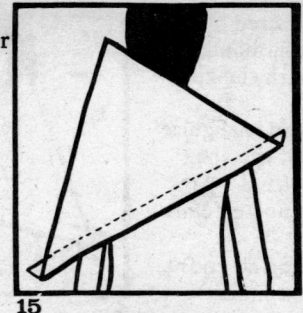
15

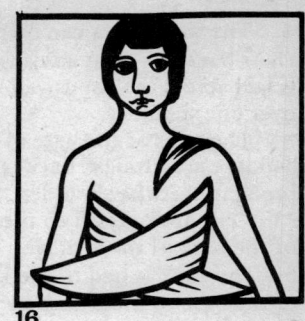
16

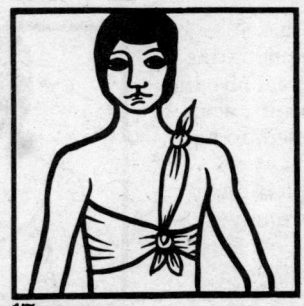
17

severe bleeding and penetrating wounds of the chest

1   When this is accompanied by internal
bleeding it can be recognised by frothy
red blood coming from the lips.

2   Treat by applying a pad to cover the
whole of the area with a firm airtight dressing.
Inserting a layer of Polythene (which can
be obtained from a Polythene bag or Polythene sheet) between the layers of dressing
will help to keep wounds airtight.

3   Fix the pad to the chest wall by firm
bandaging.

continued overleaf

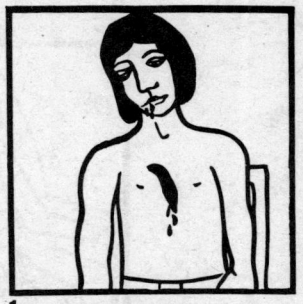
1

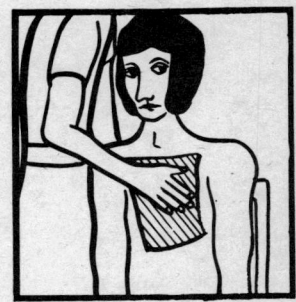
2

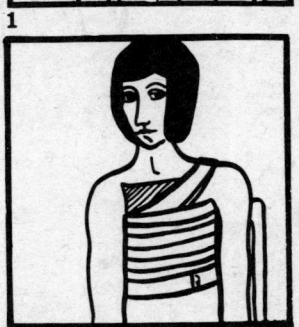
3

4   The whole area can be covered by a chest bandage. First a triangular bandage is laid across the chest wall with the apex over one shoulder.

5   The ends of the base of the triangular bandage are brought back, and the apex brought over the shoulder.

.11   The apex is tied to the knotted ends of the base of the triangle.

6   The apex is tied to the knotted ends of the base of the triangle by a short bandage.

7   Completed bandage in situ.

8   The patient with severe penetrating injury to the chest, with internal bleeding and possibly ruptured lung wants, when the dressing has been completed, to be put in a semi-upright position.

9   Breathing, pulse and respiration should be monitored very carefully.

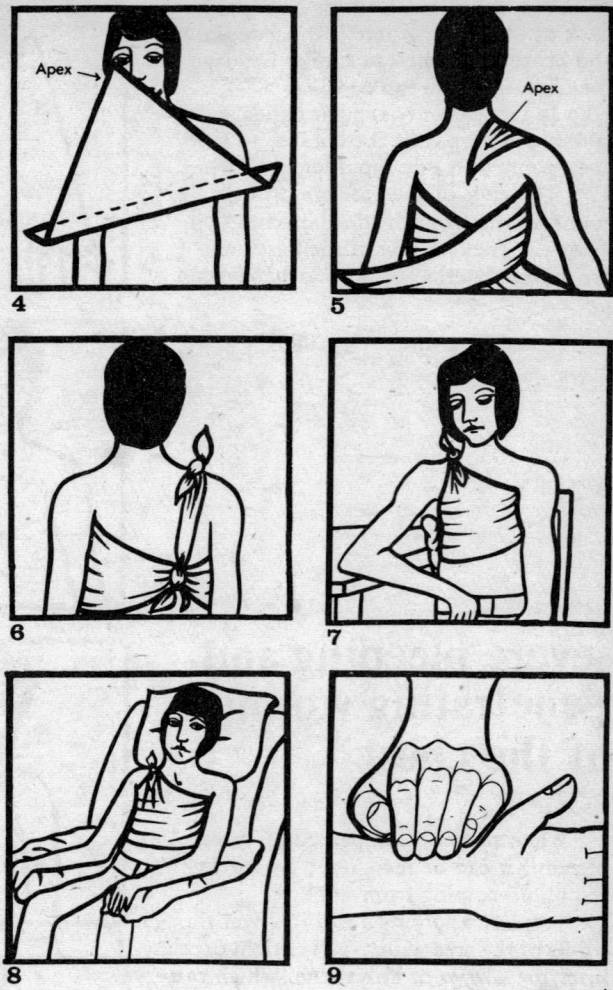

injuries to the chest where there are protruding foreign bodies such as knives or arrows

1   Do not attempt to remove the projecting material.
2   For a long splinter of wood or an arrow, management can be facilitated by cutting off any extra long piece without causing any movement of the wound.
3 to 6   The wound should then be treated as a foreign body in the chest by preparing a ring pad. Take a large square of material. Fold the material into 2-inch widths to make a bandage. Twist the bandage round on itself, and twist the ends together to make the ring pad.

continued overleaf

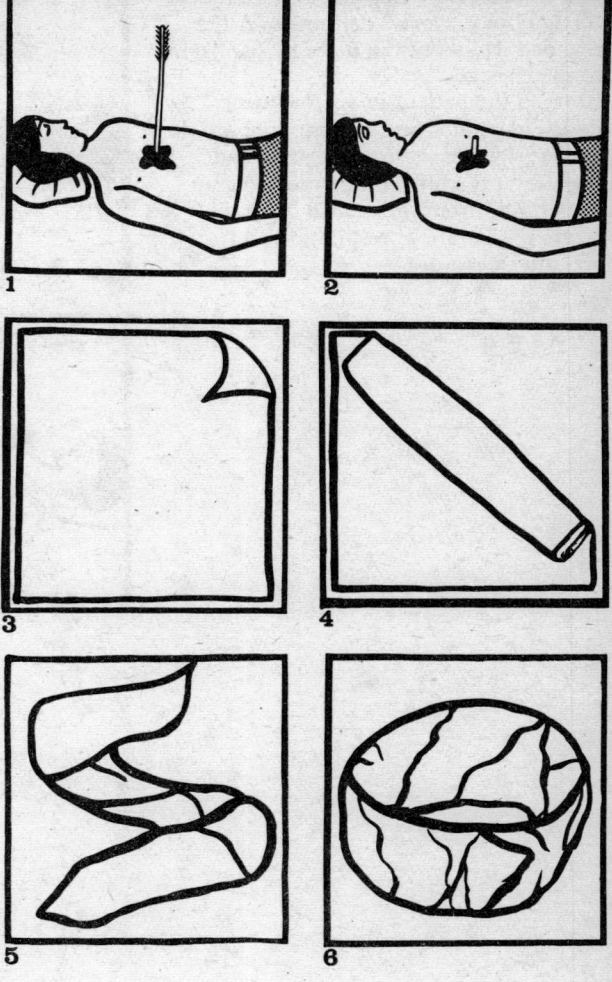

7 to 9   Place the ring pad around the foreign body. Place a dressing over the ring pad. Hold both in place by bandaging to the chest.
10 Keep the patient in a semi-sitting position, padded and comfortable. Look out for signs of internal bleeding and rupture of the lung, either coughing up fresh blood from the mouth or an increase in the rate of respiration and breathlessness.

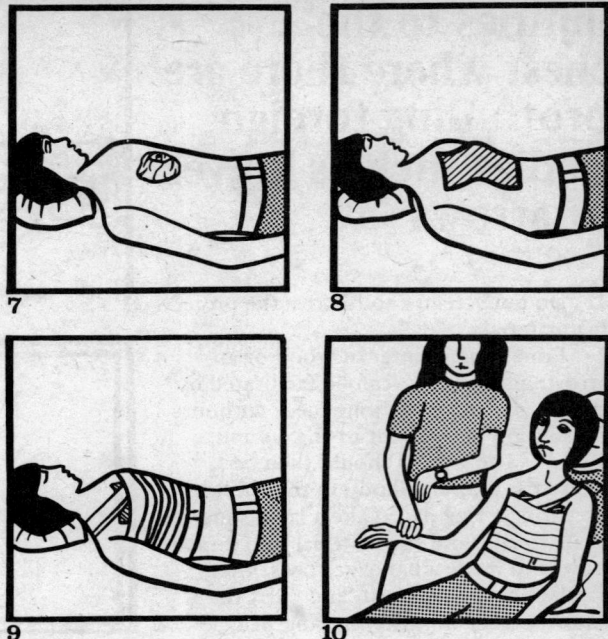

burns of the chest

Treatment of burns to the chest, be it front of the chest wall or the back, will be the principles for the treatment of all burns:
- Take away from the heat.
- Take the heat from the burn.
- Protect the burnt area from contamination and infection.

1   Where there is blistering from a burn, under no circumstances prick the blisters, they provide a sterile dressing.
2   Pour cold water over the burn.
3   Cover the burn with a paraffin gauze dressing.
4   The burnt area is covered with clean linen or sterile material to protect it from contamination and infection.
5 and 6   An ideal covering for a burn area on the chest or back is either a chest bandage adapted for the front or the back. This is made by placing a triangular bandage across the chest with the apex of the bandage over one shoulder.
7   Tie the ends of the base of the triangle round the back, then join them to the apex coming over the shoulder with a short piece of bandage.
8   A completed chest bandage covering chest and containing dressings.

continued overleaf

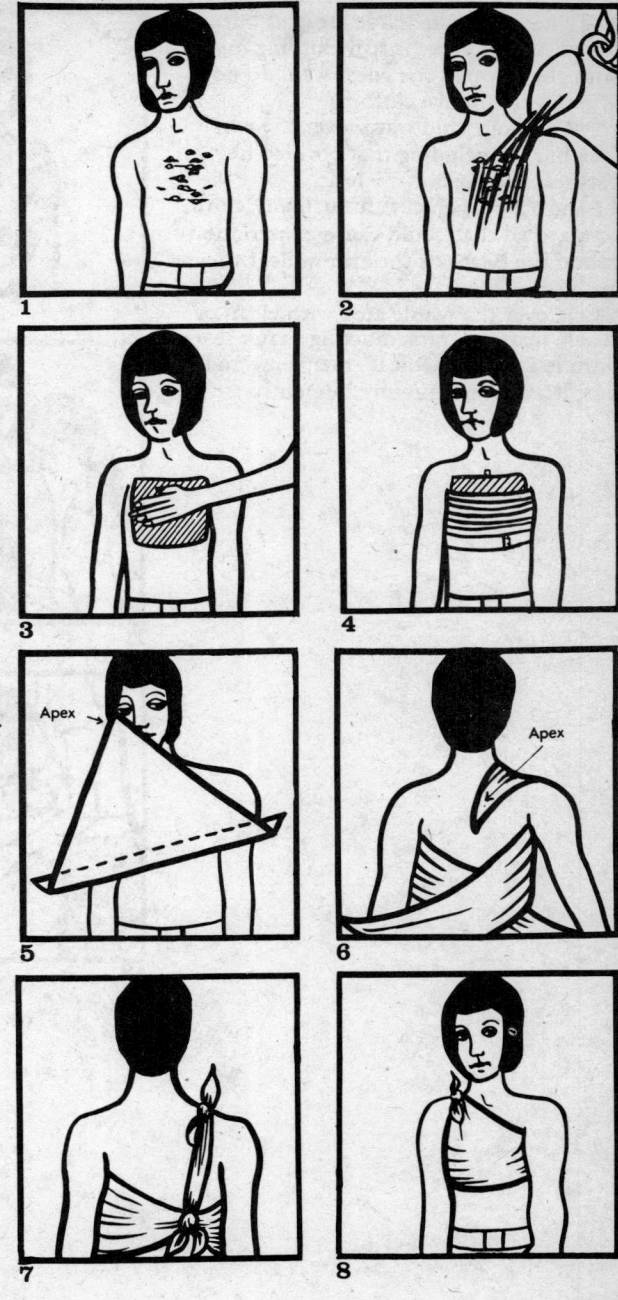

9 Where there are large areas of burns to the chest and there is still clothing mingled with the burn on the chest wall, do not attempt to remove clothing.

10 First pour cold water over the whole area burnt, including that covered by clothes, to take out the heat.

11 and 12 Then cut through any cloth or material that could cause constriction round the burns or the arm walls if they are also involved.

13 Cover the whole area with clean or sterile material, remembering that a severe burn is a major medical emergency and hospitalisation is required urgently.

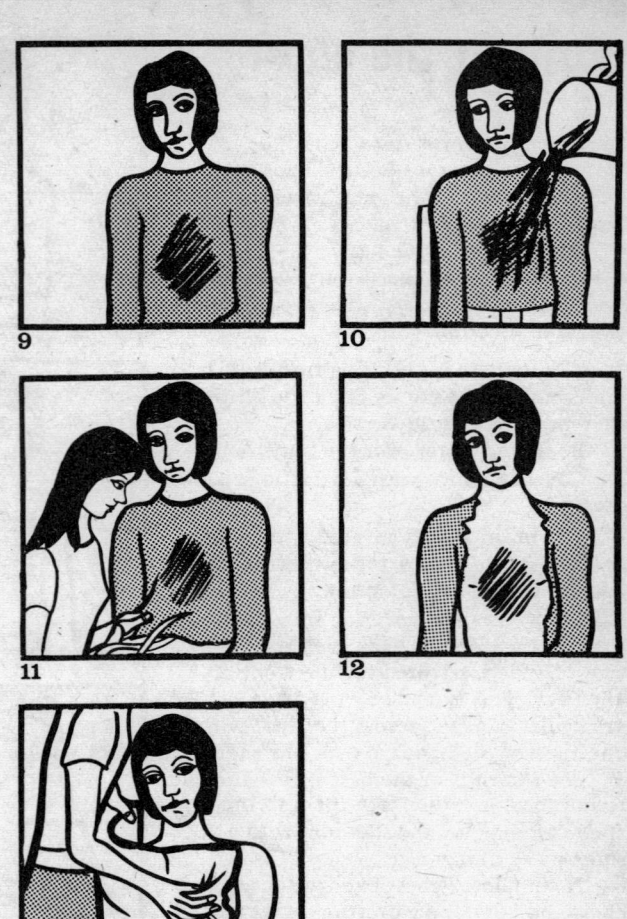

breaks in the chest

1   Suspect that there is a broken bone where either in a limb or on the body itself there is pain and deformity in the bone area. If there is pain and deformity between the neck and the shoulders, suspect that the collar bone is broken. The first aid treatment for all breaks is to reduce pain and prevent the broken ends of the bone doing further tissue damage, by immobilising the bone.

2   For broken collar bones, prevent movement round the two broken ends of the bone by making two loops of material, one to go over either shoulder and each knotted at the back.

3   Join these at the back with an encircling loop of bandage or other material, tightening as tight as possible, pulling the shoulders back and immobilising the collar bone. If available, padding placed under the bandages will prevent the tight bandage cutting into the skin.

4   Where the pain and deformity between the shoulder is at a minimum and movement is painful but not too painful, it is often sufficient just to support the arm in a sling.

5   A sling can be made by laying a bandage across the injured arm. Carry the lower end round the back under the front of the sound shoulder; tie the ends off in the hollow of the collar bone to the opposite side.

6   Tuck the point in between the forearm and the bandage, secure fold so formed to the bandage on the lower part of the upper arm.

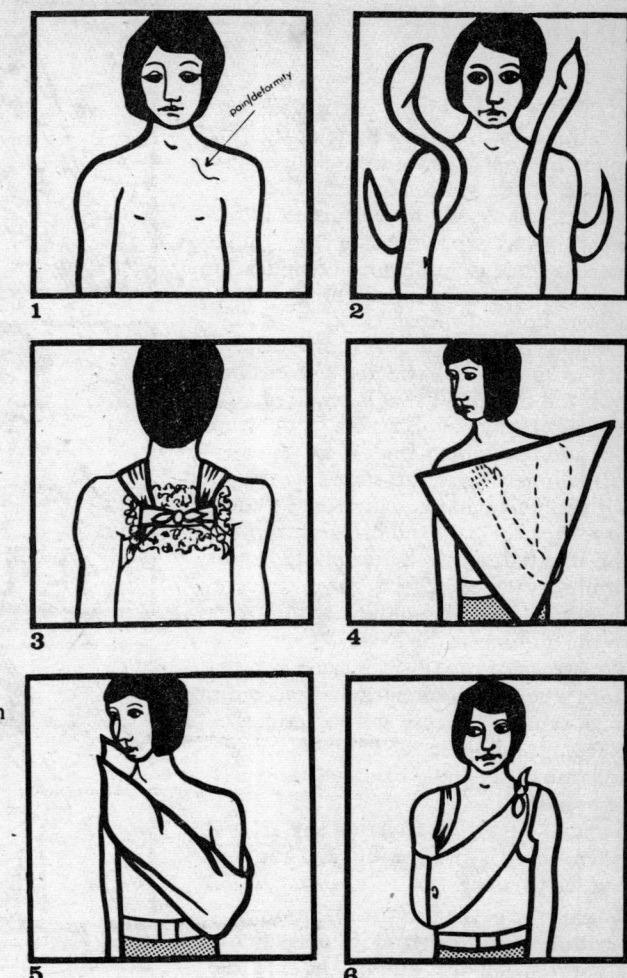

111

broken ribs

1   Where there is pain, particularly on breathing, in the breast bone or the ribs following injury or vigorous coughing, suspect that a bone is broken. The patient will usually have short, shallow breathing, as expanding the chest causes pain. If there is no obvious complication, such as rib penetrating the lung or the broken bone of the rib sticking through the skin, the patient at rest, preferably sitting up with the affected side cushioned, is all the treatment that is required.

2 to 4   If the pain is severe from broken ribs and the patient finds it extremely difficult getting about, strapping the chest with adhesive plaster can often be enough to reduce the pain and discomfort. On the affected side, adhesive plaster is put firmly on the chest from the armpit to the waist, from the midline at the front to the midline at the back.

5   Breaks of the ribs can cause complications when the broken rib has pierced the lung, causing collapse and sometimes bleeding. A hole in the lung will cause collapse of the lung, pain and shortness of breath.

6 and 7   Treat by covering any area where there is an abrasion, and apply a padded dressing.

8   Put the patient in the maximum position of comfort and if he has to be supported, support him on the side that he has been injured. Do not lie flat, but if sitting or lying, keep in a semi-upright position of 45 degrees.

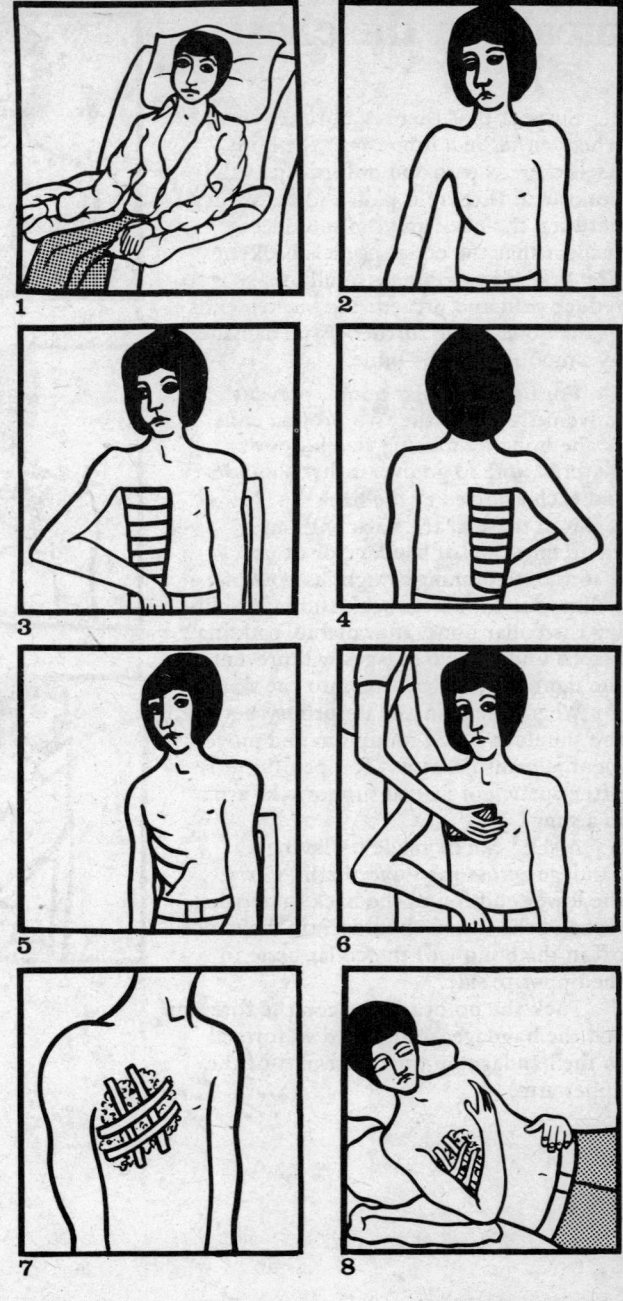

112

9 and 10   Putting the arm of the injured side in a sling does help to reduce the movement of the chest on that side, and will reduce pain.

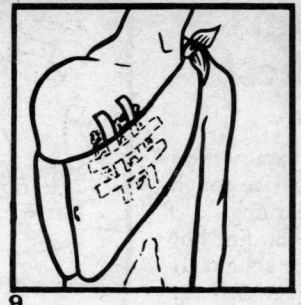

9

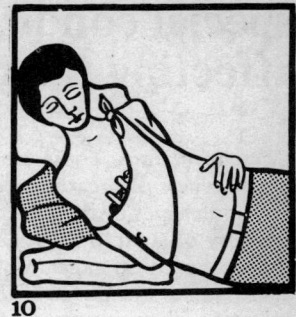

10

broken breast bone (sternum)

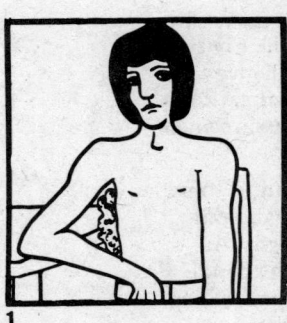

1

1   Where there is pain, both on touch and on movement of the chest, to the breast bone, suspect that the bone is broken or that the rib attachments to the breast bone are broken. The patient will have shallow breathing, as deep breathing causes further pain. If there is no obvious complication, such as a rib piercing the lungs, put the patient at rest, preferably sitting up at an angle of 45 degrees, any constricting clothing loosened, and supported at the sides. Only x-ray of this area will exclude or prove that there is bone damage.

special conditions affecting the chest

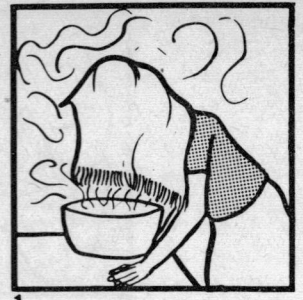

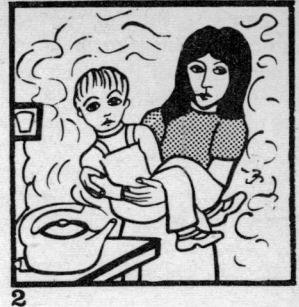

Chest Infections. These are characterised by shortness of breath, productive cough, and sometimes distress in breathing. Severity of symptoms will determine how urgently medical aid should be sought. If there is pain associated with a chest infection, then one must suspect that there is pleurisy, that the pleural cavity is involved or some other factor that needs investigation. The pleura is the skin lining inside the chest wall of the cavity which encases the lungs and will give rise to pain if there is any inflammation. The first aid treatment is to reassure and seek medical help.

1   Both adults and children can to some extent be relieved by steam inhalations while medical help is being sought. An illness common in children is the condition called Croup, where there is swelling in the main breathing tube, causing them distress and for them to make a characteristic sound similar to that of the barking of a seal. Where pain is associated with chest infections, a hot water bottle applied to the painful area will, to some extent, relieve symptoms.

2   For croup and obstructive breathing, let the patient breathe in steam. For the older child let him breathe over a bowl of boiling water with a towel over his head, catching the water vapour. For the younger child who may not co-operate enough to do this, an electric kettle boiling in the kitchen, filling the room with steam, will probably be enough. Do not let the child get too near to the nozzle of the kettle. To bring up phlegm, the sipping of hot drinks is often very beneficial.

coronary thrombosis and heart attack

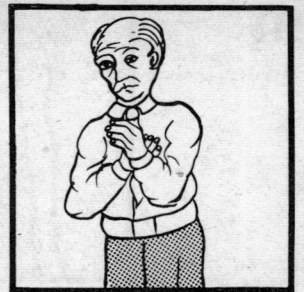

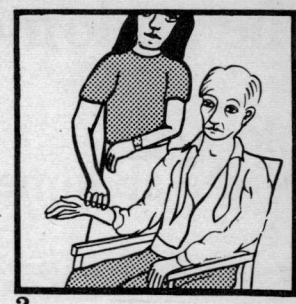

1   Coronary thrombosis may be recognised by the onset of a severe constricting pain under the breast bone. The patient may be shocked, grey-looking, and short of breath, and the pain may radiate down the left arm and up into the neck.

2   The patient must be reassured, put at rest, restrictive clothing loosened, and medical aid sent for. While awaiting medical aid the attendant should keep a check on the strength and volume of the patient's pulse, rate of respiration and general level of sensibility.

3   If the patient's condition should deteriorate and he loses consciousness, he should be put in the coma/recovery position, with a continual check on the pulse and respiration, being prepared to give artificial resuscitation if breathing or heart stops.

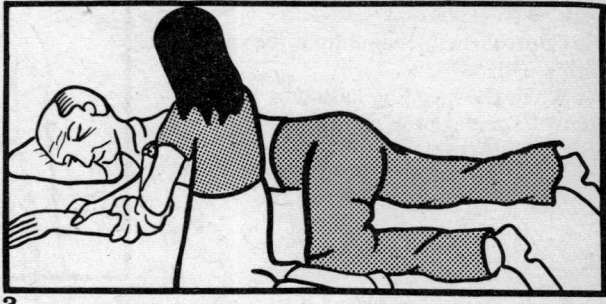

4   A heart attack, other than a coronary thrombosis, usually occurs in patients with long standing heart disease who, for a variety of reasons, have gone into failure. They are characterised by blueness of the lips, shortness of breath, engorgement of the neck veins, and possible swelling of the ankles. The patient should be put in the cardiac position, i.e. at an angle of 45 degrees, half sitting up (this is the position of the body in which the heart has to do the least work), reassured, made comfortable, and restrictive clothing loosened, and medical aid sought, the attendant keeping a check on pulse rate and general condition so that a clear account can be given to the medical aid when it arrives as to whether the patient's condition is deteriorating, improving, or staying the same.

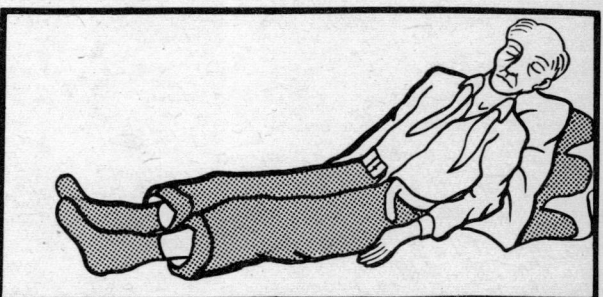

the abdomen

bleeding of the abdomen

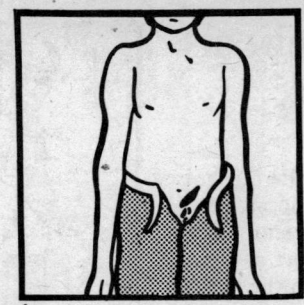

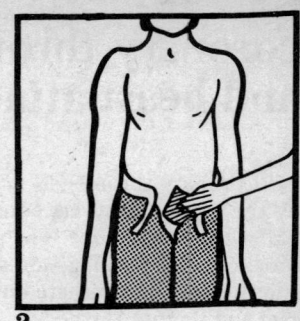

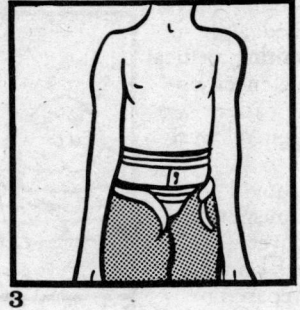

1 *Superficial cuts to the abdomen and lower back,* where the injury has not penetrated right through the abdominal wall.

2 Control the bleeding by direct pressure with a pad.

3 When the bleeding has come under control, bandage the pad firmly into position.

4 For *penetrating wounds* of the
abdomen, stab wounds, etc., where there
is no foreign body . . .
5 . . . cover the wound with a pad . . .
6 . . . and apply a bandage. Keep a check
on the patient's condition for signs of
internal bleeding. The signs that there may
be bleeding inside would be an increase
in the pulse rate, decrease in the pulse
volume, rapid breathing, and a pale and
anxious-looking patient.

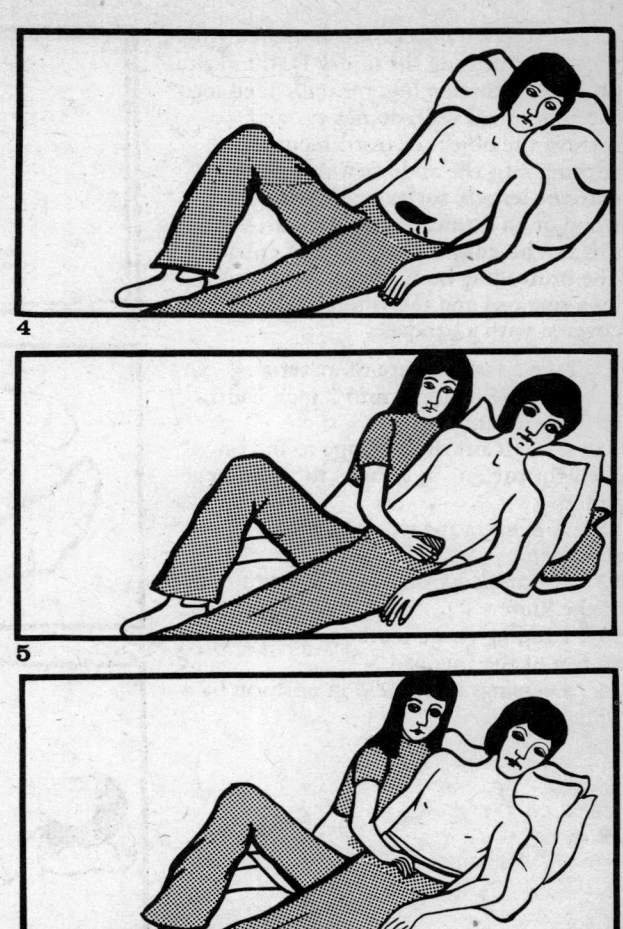

4

5

6

For *stab wounds to the abdomen* where the object causing the injury is still in situ or where a foreign body is imbedded into the abdominal wall, do not try and remove the object or instrument that is sticking into the **abdomen**. If it is of extreme length, for example a piece of wood or an arrow, to facilitate dressing this can be cut near its point of entry. The protruding body should be protected by a ring pad and the whole area then covered with a bandage.

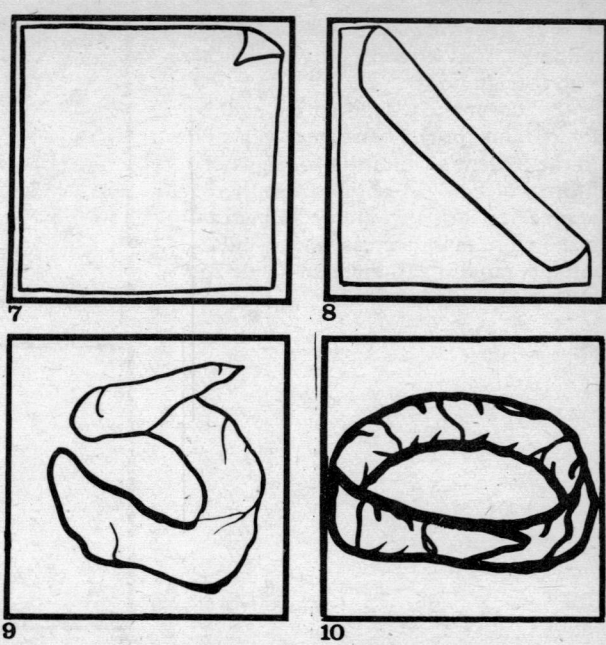

7   Take a large square of material.
8   Fold the material into 2 inch widths to make a bandage.
9 and 10   Curl the bandage round on itself for tucking in corners to make ring pad.
11   A penetrating wound of the abdomen.
12   A ring pad around the point of entry of the knife.
13   Padding tissue placed around the knife on top of the ring pad.
14   Dressings being held in position by a wide bandage.

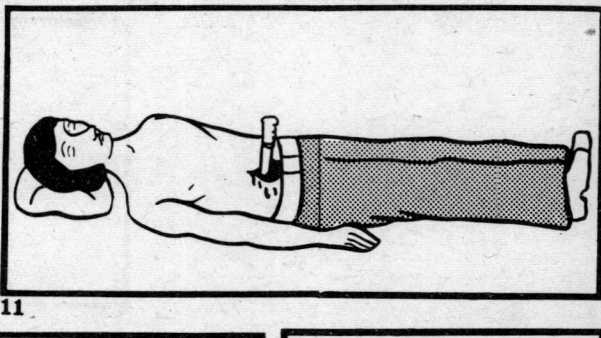

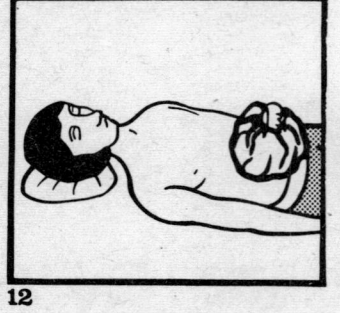
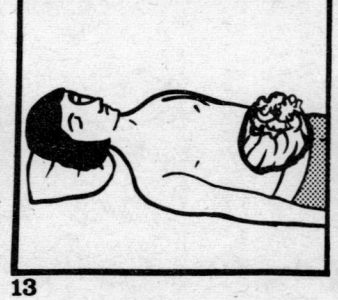
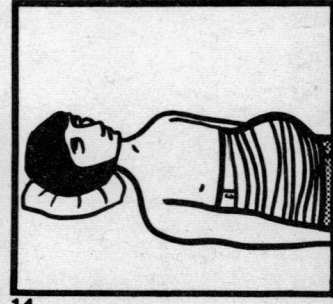

15 and 16 In the case of an arrow wound or something similar, the patient may be more easily transportable if the arrow shaft is cut off just above the skin. Follow with dressing sequence 7 to 13.

The attendant, as well as treating the wound, must keep a check on the patient's condition for deterioration, signs of internal bleeding, which are characterised by a rise in the pulse rate, sweating, paleness, shortness of breath, and a generalised state of apprehension.

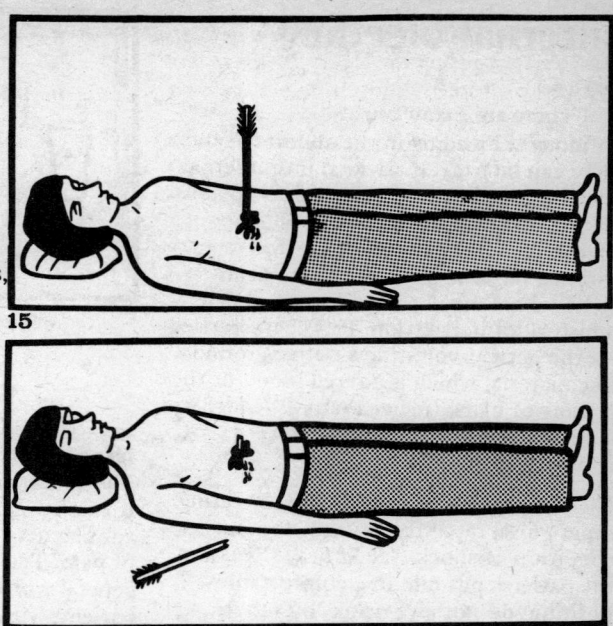

15

16

internal bleeding

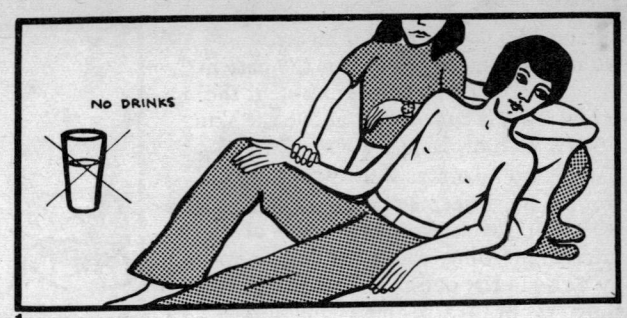

There are many causes
of internal bleeding in the abdomen, and
they can be roughly divided into internal
bleeding where there has been no obvious
injury, and internal bleeding following
an injury. The commonest site for
internal bleeding is from the stomach
where there may or may not have been
a history of indigestion. It is characterised
by the patient vomiting a coffee-ground
like material which is altered blood or the
passing of black (melena) stools, which are
characterised by their black, tarry
consistency.

1   The patient is apprehensive, sweating,
rapid pulse, rapid respiration, and in a
condition of shock (see *Shock*). Reassure
the patient, put him in a comfortable
position, do not give drinks by mouth,
seek medical aid and in the meantime
keep a check on pulse, respiration and
general condition so a full report can be
given to medical aid when it arrives.

Internal bleeding following injury is an
extremely dangerous situation, and first
aid attendants must be constantly on the
lookout for it. The spleen or liver, or
intestines, could be ruptured, and bleeding
can sometimes be so insidious as to be
missed. But if, following a blow to the
abdomen, the patient is unwell, his
general condition deteriorates, there is
sweating and his pulse rate goes up,
suspect there may be internal bleeding.
The abdomen may or may not be tender.
It can be rigid or have a doughy-like
consistency. There may be certain areas
of pain. The main indications are the
general worsening of the condition of the
patient, with sweating, increased pulse
rate, and presentation of shock (see
Shock). This is a medical emergency,
and the patient must be got to medical
aid at the earliest opportunity. Put him
in a position of optimum rest and comfort
(which is lying, supported at an angle of
about 45 degrees). Do not give him drinks
by mouth, reassure him, and keep a check
on his general condition so a report can
be given to medical aid when it arrives.

*If fluids by mouth are given, it might
necessitate the delay of a life-saving
operation.*

burns
to the abdomen

1   Follow the first principles for treating
burns. Take away from the heat, take
the heat away from the burn, then protect
burn from contamination and infection
by covering.

2   For *small superficial burns*, pour cold
water over the burnt area. When possible,
treat by applying paraffin gauze.

3 and 4   Cover dressed burn with either
sterile or clean bandage or material to
protect.

5   *Severe burns to the abdomen.* Where
large areas of the abdomen are burnt,
this is a medical emergency.

6   Take the heat out of the burn by
pouring cold water over the burn.

7   Do not attempt to take clothing
material off burnt areas. Cut through
singly any clothing that might obstruct
both round the abdomen and going down,
and including the legs.

8   Cover the whole area with clean or
sterile material and transport to hospital
for treatment. The severely burnt can be
given fluids by mouth, but no solids.

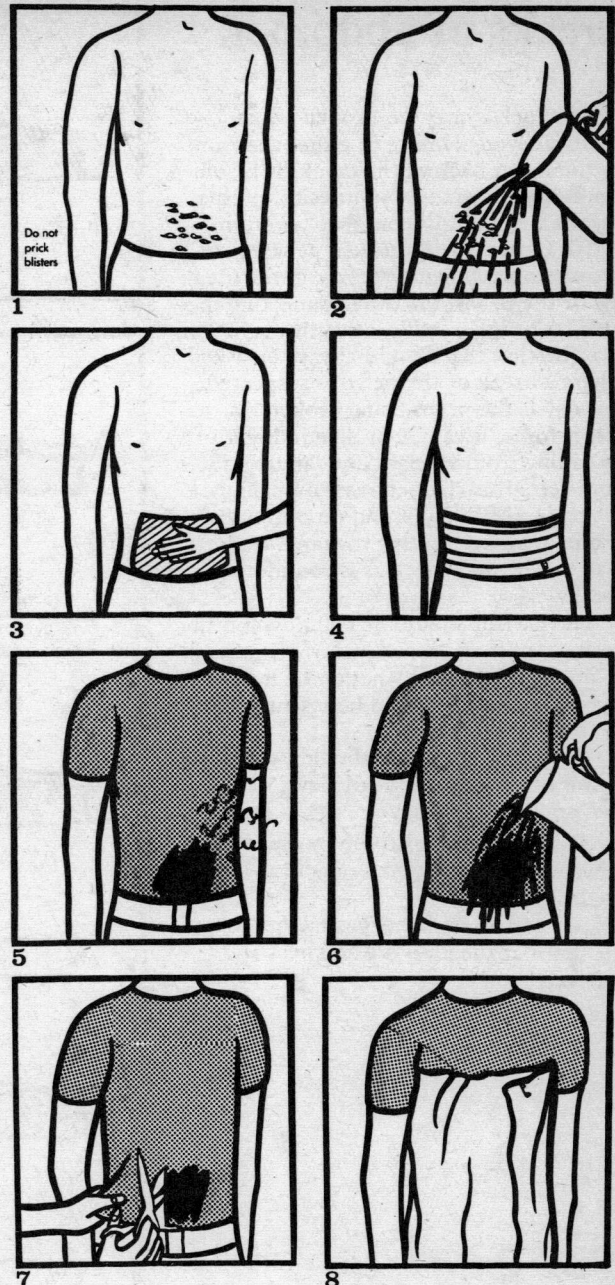

breaks of abdomen

The pelvis may be broken when there is severe damage to either the front or the lower back of the trunk. It is sometimes complicated by injuries to internal organs and a not uncommon symptom is that patients with broken pelvises are unable to pass their water as, in the breaking of the pelvis, the tube connecting the bladder to the outside is cut through. This is a question that should always be asked where a break of the pelvis is suspected. As well as the pelvis being broken by direct force, it can be broken indirectly by falling from a height and landing on both feet. It is characterised by pain in the region of the hips and on movement and pain on attempting to stand. There may not be deformity as is common in most breaks.

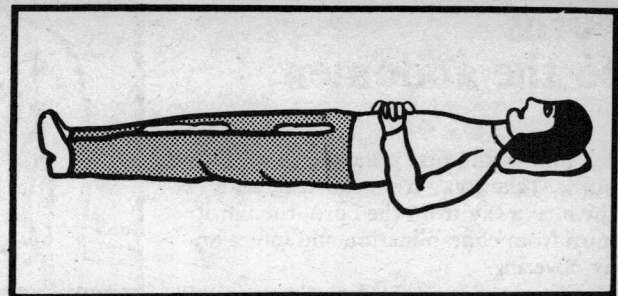

1   The patient should be laid down in the position of maximum comfort. He should be questioned about whether he has passed water and should be instructed not to try and pass water.

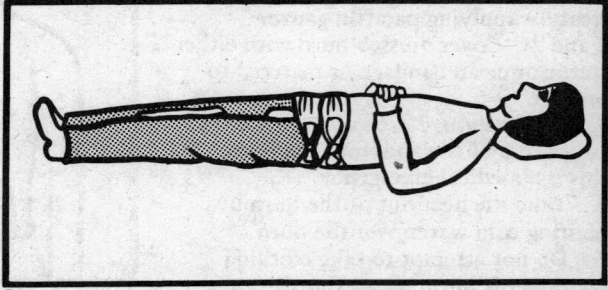

2   Two wide bandages should be applied round the pelvis, one at the level of the hips and one just above.

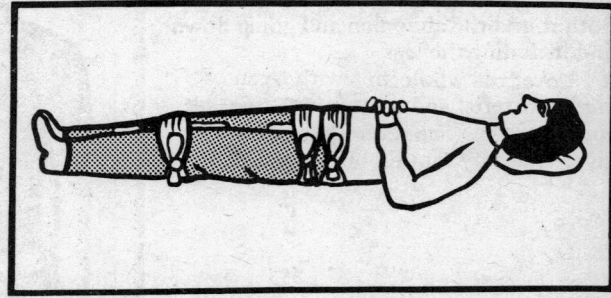

3   If the patient has to be transported, movement is decreased by padding between the legs . . .

4   . . . and apply bandages further down the limbs at the level of the knees and the feet.

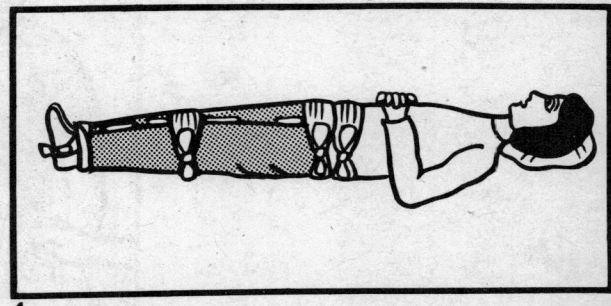

breaks to the spine (at the lower part of the back)

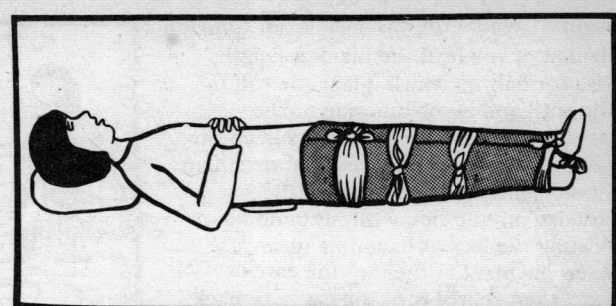

1

Suspect that there may be a break in the spinal bones if a patient has had direct damage to the lower back by a blow or a heavy fall on the buttocks or the feet. If there is pain and tenderness in this area, suspect that the spine may be injured. The most important aspect is to prevent damage to the spinal cord. The spinal cord may be already damaged and can manifest itself by causing loss of power and sensation (feeling) in the legs. The first aid attendant's duty is to prevent movement in the area of the break. If possible, leave in the situation as found and pad the whole area so that there is no pressure on one particular part of the back. Do not move the patient or turn him over.

If, for example, the patient was in the middle of a motorway and had to be moved to a place of safety, as many hands as possible, first having padded the limbs and cavities to prevent any movement or bearing down of body weight, should then move the patient in this position. If the patient is unconscious in this situation, do not put him into the coma/recovery position as this could cause further damage to the spine. The patient is always best left in the position found when this is possible, and padded to prevent any movement or unequal down of body weight.

1 Where he has to be transported, broad bandages should be tied round the thighs, knees and ankles, moving the patient as little as possible while they are being applied.

continued overleaf

2 and 3 Where the casualty is not lying on a blanket or rug, roll the blanket lengthwise for half its width, place the roll in line with and along one side of the casualty. Whilst two attendants keep the body in firm control, the other attendants should gently and slowly turn the casualty on one side without bending or twisting the legs or back in any way. Move the blanket then up the casualty's back, then gently turn the casualty back over the roll of blanket on the opposite side. Unroll the blanket and turn the casualty on his back.

4 and 5 When the patient is on the blanket, with the blanket taut and firmly supporting the body, the patient can be moved on to a stretcher without changing his position.

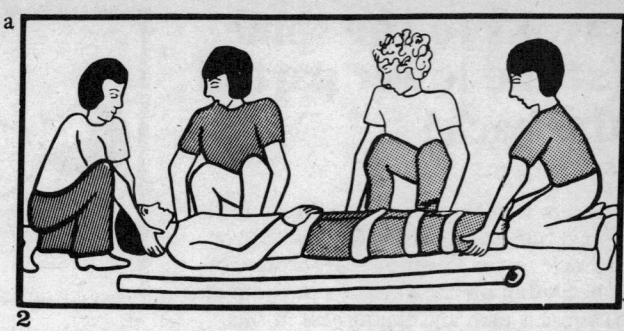

2

3

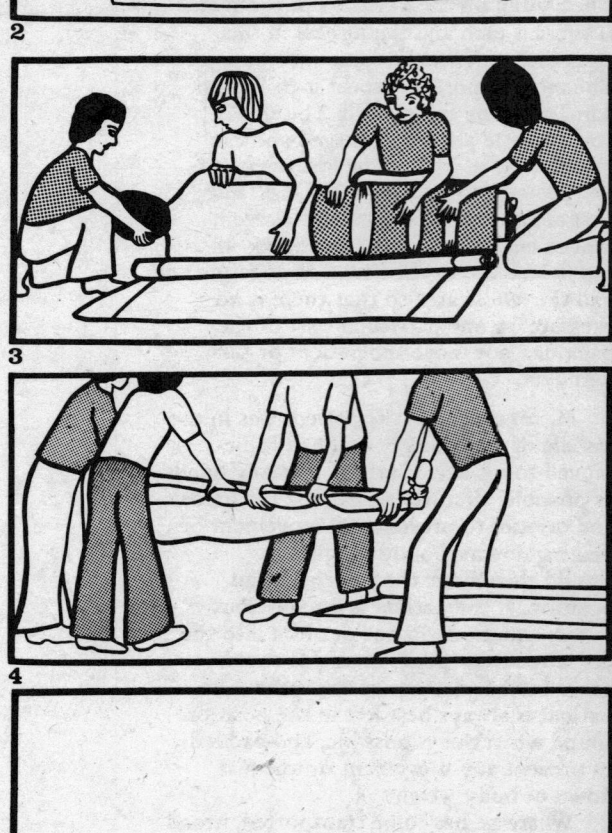

4

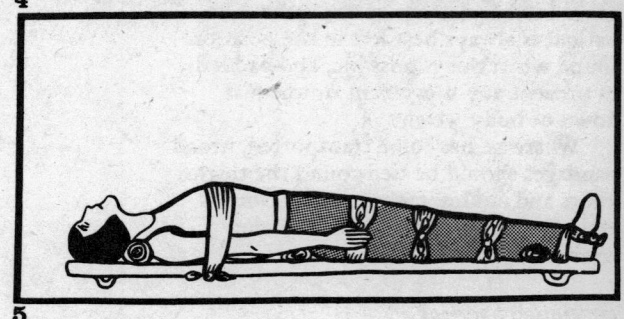

5

special conditions affecting the abdomen

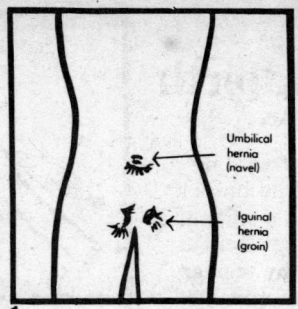
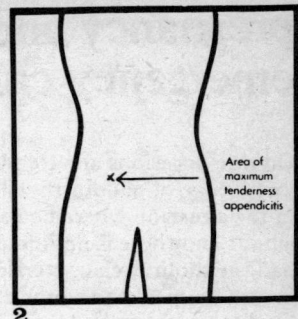

Hernias. Hernias occur when the abdominal contents are squeezed through areas of the abdominal wall where there is muscular weakness. There are three main sites. One is the navel and the other two are the groins. There can also be a hernia resulting in a weakness left by an operation scar.

1   Where a hernia becomes strangulated, twisted, it will be painful and tense and the patient will vomit, and urgent medical help is required. A first aid attendant finding this situation where a patient has a tender, painful hernia and is vomiting, should not attempt to push the hernia back as the contents of the hernia may have become gangrenous, but should seek urgent medical help. Do not give drinks as this might delay the speed of an urgent operation.

The acute abdomen. The acute abdomen is a situation where some abdominal mishap has occurred that requires urgent surgery. Pain and tenderness of the abdominal wall, associated with vomiting, is an indication that this has taken place. If the onset of the pain is sudden and the abdominal wall is rigid and board-like, then it is probable that there has been a perforation of the stomach contents into the abdomen.

2   *Appendicitis* must be suspected when there is pain, tenderness and resistance in the right lower side of the abdomen, possibly associated with a slight rise of temperature and with nausea and vomiting. This requires instant hospitalisation.

Appendicitis can present in many other ways, and the duty of the first aid attendant in the presence of abdominal pain where there is tenderness on pressure to the abdomen is to obtain an expert opinion. There are many other conditions that can simulate both appendicitis and perforation of the stomach, all of which require urgent hospitalisation and the first aider's duty is not to diagnose but to refer.

Tubal Pregnancies. One abdominal condition that requires the most urgent medical treatment is where a pregnancy starts in one of the tubes leading to the womb instead of the womb, and the tube bursts, causing bleeding inside the abdomen. Suspect this might have occurred when a female patient is overdue three to four weeks from her expected period time suddenly collapses with abdominal pain, at the same time having a small loss of vaginal blood.

Miscarriage. Any bleeding following the commencement of pregnancy must be considered as a threatened abortion. If there are rhythmic pains with the bleeding, then it is almost certain that a miscarriage will take place. Painless bleeding, however, may settle down with rest. In both cases medical aid should be summoned or notified.

pregnancy and emergency childbirth

On rare occasions an attendant with no knowledge of childbirth will find himself in the situation where he has a woman in labour and there is no immediate help at hand. Labour is characterised by regular contractions of the womb, accompanied by discomfort to the patient in labour.

1   The first aid attendant should not try and interfere in the course of the pregnancy. If delivery is imminent, i.e. the baby's head is beginning to appear at the vaginal opening, then the patient should not be moved as birth is likely to take place in the next few minutes. The patient should be either on her back, knees bent with feet wide apart . . .

2   . . . or in the left lateral position, that is to say, on one side with the uppermost leg bent and raised to clear the emerging head of the new baby. Unless the attendant has some knowledge of delivery, he should not attempt to intertere with the delivery of the head.

3   Once the head has been delivered, he should feel behind the neck to see if the umbilical cord is present. Its situation there will put it in the danger of being obstructing to delivery and the baby's breathing, so it should be pulled over the head of the baby towards the face so as not to obstruct or impede the baby in any way. While the head is protruding from the vagina, before delivery of the body, the attendant should clean out any mucus or fluid from the baby's mouth, gently, with some clean, dry linen.

4   Once the baby has been delivered, if it is not breathing, the attendant should support the baby by the feet, with the head in a downward position, allowing it to drain off any fluids, and check

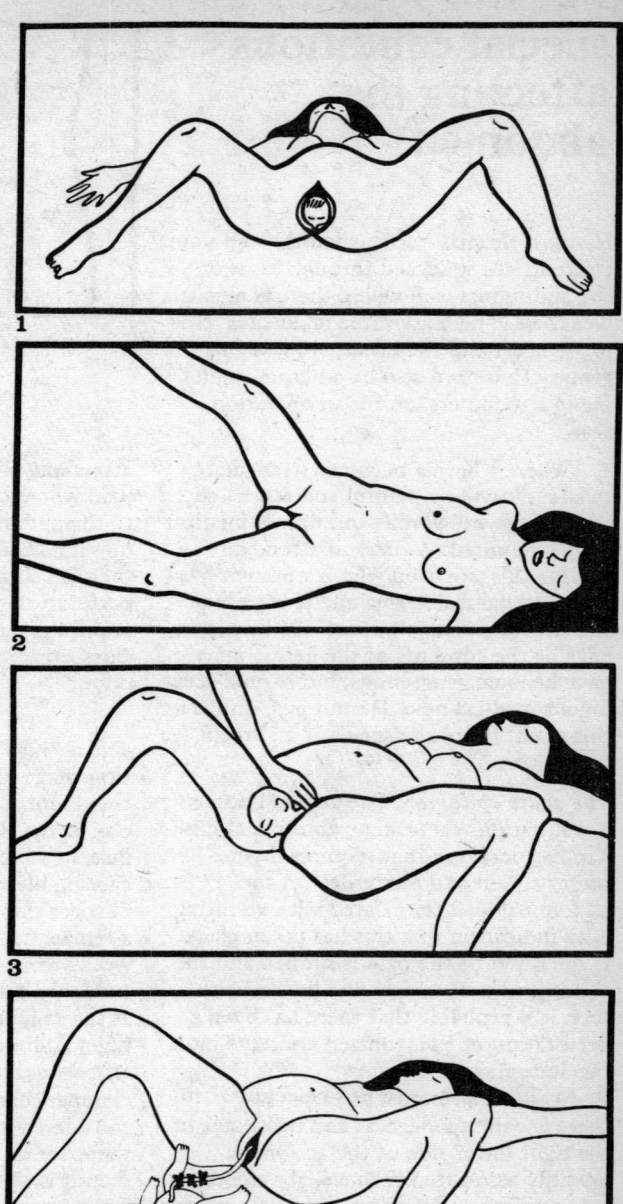

that the mouth is not being obstructed by fluid or any other material. If help is not at hand, the umbilical cord should be divided 6 inches from the baby, three knots should be tied in the cord with string (preferably sterile string if this is possible).

5   Then the cord should be cut through with a pair of scissors between the second and third ligature, counting the ligature nearest the baby as ligature number one.

6   The baby should then be wrapped in clean linen and given to the mother.

7   The afterbirth will follow within 15 to 20 minutes of the delivery of the baby. She should be encouraged to push if she feels the womb contracting, but unless the attendant has some previous knowledge of the management of childbirth, he should not try and extract the afterbirth himself. Only in a situation after the delivery of the afterbirth where there is severe bleeding from the vagina should the attendant try and reduce the flow of blood by stimulating the womb to contract. If the bleeding is exceptionally severe after the delivery of the afterbirth the attendant should feel for the top of the womb by placing his hand on the stomach just below the navel. Having found this rounded lump, he should rub it with moderate firmness until he feels it harden under his hand and the bleeding stops.

   The afterbirth should be carefully wrapped up so that it can be later inspected by medical help to ensure that it is complete.

8   After delivery, wrap mother up warm and give her a hot sweet drink.

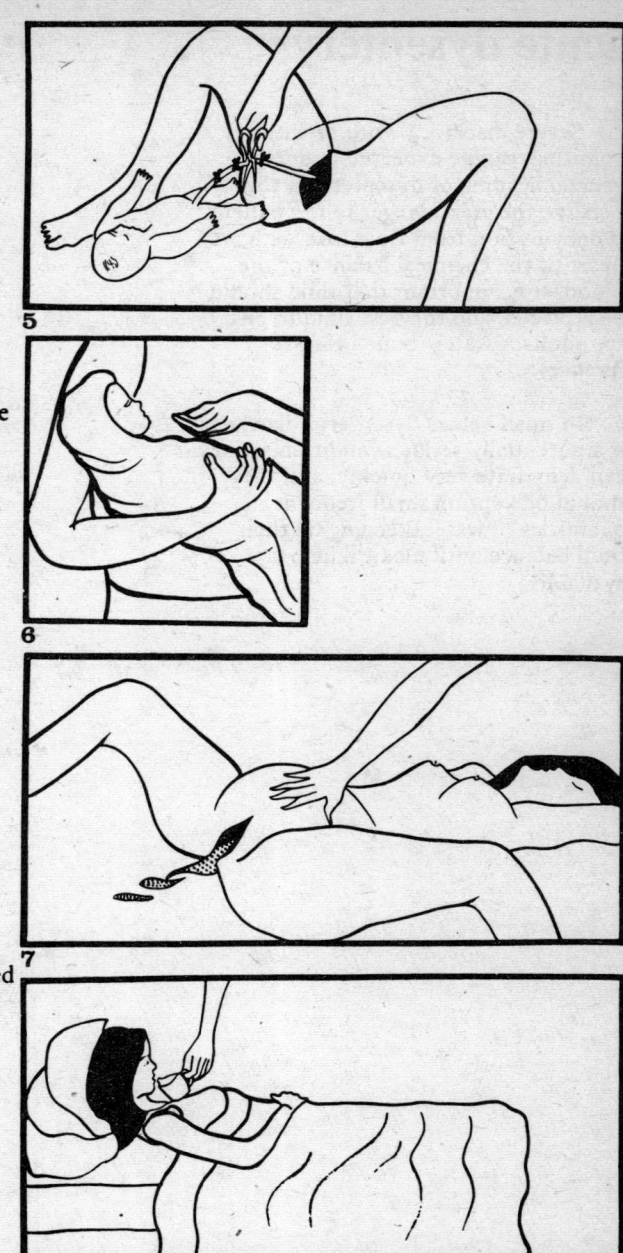

acute dysentery

Severe diarrhoea, with or without vomiting, can be expected under the general heading of dysentery. If this persists, the great danger to the patient is dehydration from fluid loss, with an upset of the chemical balance of the blood. It is important that fluid should be replaced, and the best fluid to give for adults is water (boiled for preference).

In small babies dysentery (diarrhoea) is a potentially serious condition as they can dehydrate very quickly, and they should be kept on small frequent quantities of water, keeping up their fluid balance until medical help is available.

resuscitation

Resuscitation (artificial respiration) is required when a patient, for one of many reasons, has either obstructed breathing or has stopped breathing, or where the heart has stopped beating. It is the attendant's responsibility to restart and maintain life until expert help is obtained.

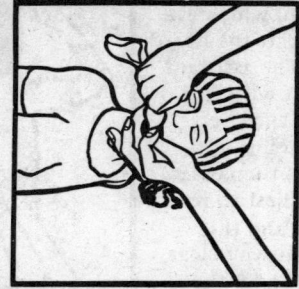

1   In commencing any form of resuscitation, the first step always is to see that the main airway is patent, i.e. that the mouth is not blocked with vomit, saliva, false teeth, etc., and this must be cleared out before resuscitation can commence. The principle aimed at is to put air into the lungs when the patient is unable to do this himself and stimulate the heart to start it beating again if it has stopped. Failure of respiration (breathing) is noted by cessation of movement of the chest and blue-ish discolouration of the lips, fingers, ears and other peripheral parts of the body.

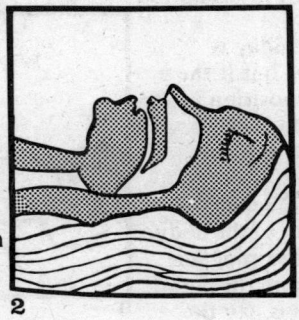

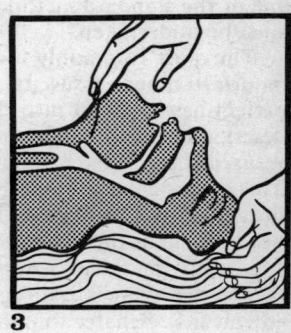

2   There are many methods of resuscitation. The first is to make sure that there is not some mechanical obstruction in the mouth or upper throat that is causing the breathing difficulties.

3   When this has been eliminated the second step is seeing whether change of the position of the head will open up the airway. It is often sufficient just to lift the chin of the patient to relieve breathing obstruction.

To resuscitate the unconscious non-breathing patient, first see that the airway is clear, then use one of the several methods available of getting air into the lungs and restarting the heart. The author believes that prior to starting any of the standard methods of resuscitation, the patient should have his airway inspected, be laid on his face with his hands folded across in front of the head, face turned to one side. The attendant then gives the back a hard
continued overleaf

thump with the flat of his palm, which can help dislodge obstructions, restart the heart or even stimulate respiration. The assistant kneels at the side of the patient with the flat of his hand on the back of the chest and presses firmly on the chest, but not putting his body weight into it, then eases off the pressure, allowing the chest to re-expand. If, after two pressures and the thump into the back with the airway clear, respiration has not been established, then one of the standard methods of resuscitation must be undertaken.

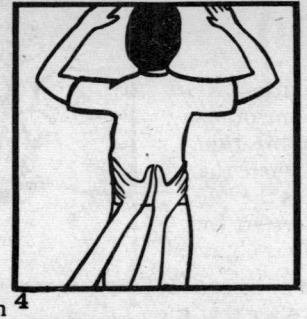

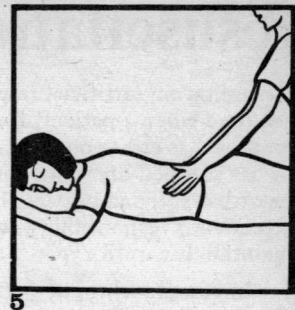

4   5

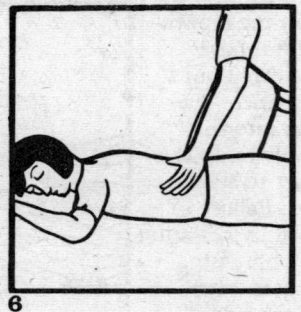

6

The most commonly used today is mouth-to-mouth resuscitation, but if the patient has been put into the position as described, then the older method of resuscitation, called Schafers, can be used. This is particularly useful in cases of drowning, and in the case of drowning the head should be the lowest point of the body. If possible, get the patient on a sloping sur-face so that there is drainage from the mouth downwards. Schafer's method is, lay the patient face downwards with the head turned to one side and the arms folded on either side of the head. Make sure there is no obstruction to the mouth and that the airway is clean. The attendant kneels on one side of the patient facing his head, the hands are placed under the small of the back of the lower ribs, the attendant sits back then so as not to put his body weight on the chest, then the body is slowly swung forward from the knees, keeping the arms straight and the hands in position, all the time maintaining a steady pressure. Keep this pressure on for two seconds and then relax. A rhythmical pressure is then established in the follow-ing sequence—
(a) Swing forward.
(b) Apply pressure.

(c) Release pressure.
(d) Rest back with pressure off.
These movements must be carried out 10 to 12 times a minute.

4   Position of hands for resuscitation.
5   Arms should be straight with the hands on the small of the back, thumbs almost touching, with no pressure on the patient. Count three seconds, then swing slowly forward from the knees, keeping the arms straight and the hands in place all the time.
6   The attendant's weight without extra exertion should bear down on the patient for two seconds before relaxing in the position in figure 5.

mouth-to-mouth resuscitation

This can be used on all age groups except where there is severe injury to the face or mouth or if vomiting interferes with resuscitation.

1   Lay the patient on his back, ensure that the airway is patent by cleaning out the mouth. Loosen clothing at the neck and waist.

2   Support the nape of the neck and press top of the head so that it is tilted backwards, pushing the chin upwards.

3   If the patient does not start to breathe, with the chin still pushed up and the head tilted backward, pinch the patient's nose, take a deep breath, seal your lips round the patient's mouth, blow into the lungs and watch the chest rise.

4   Stop blowing when the chest has risen, remove your mouth and watch the chest fall.

5 and 6   This can be continued at the normal rate of breathing until breathing is restored in an infant or child it is important to remember to breathe very gently or damage can be done. If the patient's heart is not beating, strike the chest smartly on the left lower part of the breast bone; if there is no response, start striking rhythmically for 10 seconds, feeling the pulse for evidence of re-starting the heart. If no pulse felt, proceed to external cardiac compression. (See *When the Heart has Stopped*, page 134).

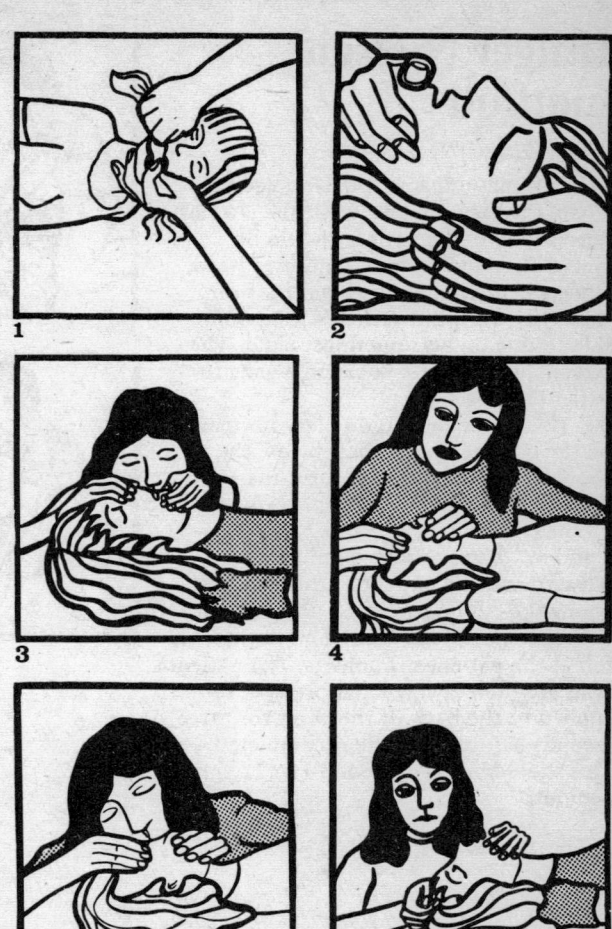

Holger Nielsen method

1   This method is particularly useful where the face is damaged or the jaw has been broken. The patient should be placed face downwards, arms over head, elbows bent so that one hand rests on the other, with the patient's head on one side resting on his uppermost hand. The attendant should be kneeling, facing the patient's head.

2   The attendant should place his hands on the patient's back chest below the shoulder blades and rock forwards with the elbows straight, exerting steady pressure on the chest.

3 and 4   The pressure should then be released and the patient's arms held just below the elbow and lifted upwards and backwards until resistance and tension are felt at the patient's shoulders. The patient's arms are then lowered and pressure re-applied to the back of the chest for three seconds before the cycle is completed. This should be carried out 10 to 12 times a minute.

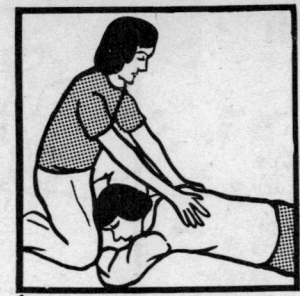
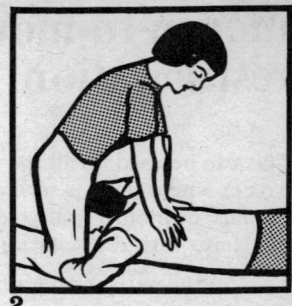
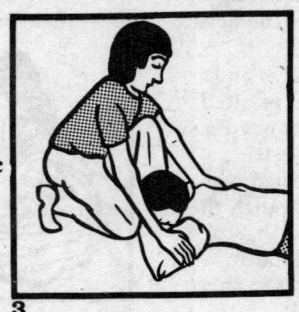
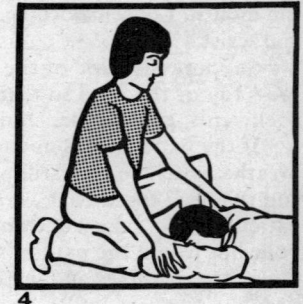

Silvester method

1   This is again particularly useful for patients with facial injuries who cannot have mouth-to-mouth resuscitation. Lie the patient on his back on a firm surface, padding of rolled material, blankets, coats, etc., under shoulders. Check that the mouth and airway are clear and let the head drop back over the folded padding. Cross the patient's wrists over the lower part of the chest.

2   The attendant should then rock forward and press down on the patient's chest, holding the patient's wrists.

3 and 4   This should be maintained for three seconds, then the pressure released and the patient's arms brought backwards and outwards before being folded and returned to the lower chest. The attendant should establish a rhythm and it should be repeated 10 to 12 times a minute.

5   All forms of artificial respiration should be kept going until respiration starts. When this does so, patient should be put in the coma/recovery position, lying on one side with the lower leg extended and the upper leg bent, the lower arm behind the back and the upper arm in front of the face. The attendant should check that the airway is clear and that regular breathing is maintained.

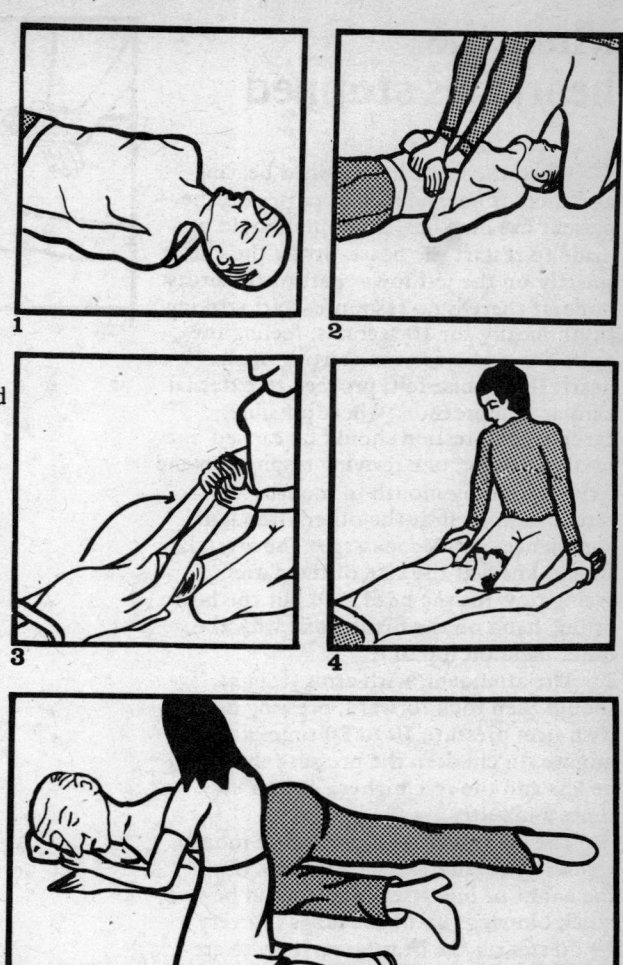

when the heart has stopped

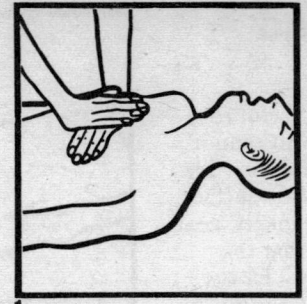
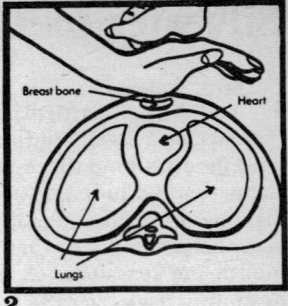

1   When the heart has stopped beating
and there is no evidence of pulse and the
patient has blue lips, attempts should be
made to restart the heart. Strike the chest
smartly on the left lower part of the breast
bone. If there is no response, start striking
rhythmically for 10 seconds, feeling the
pulse for evidence of re-starting of the
heart. If no pulse felt, proceed to external
cardiac compression. Where possible,
cardiac compression should be carried out
by two people, one reviving respiration and
oxygenation by mouth-to-mouth
resuscitation whilst the other attendant
commences cardiac massage. The attendant
should kneel at the side of the patient,
facing towards the head, and put the heel
of one hand on the breastbone with the
other hand on top of it.
2   The attendant, with arms straight,
should then rock forward, pressing down
with firm pressure 40 to 50 times a
minute. In children the pressure should
be less and the rate higher — 60 to 80
times a minute.
     The combination of mouth-to-mouth
resuscitation and cardiac massage, if in
the hands of one attendant, should be two
quick blowings up of the lungs to every
14 presses on the heart area; if there are
two first aiders, one deep lung inflation
should be undertaken for every five
heart compressions. Look for recovery
with an improvement of colour in the
patient and pulsations in the arteries of
the neck.

fits and convulsions

convulsions

1   Convulsions occur most commonly in young children and are associated usually with a raised temperature. A child may have several of these attacks during his early years but the vast majority grow out of them without further trouble. The child may be twitching and squirming, with rigidity of limbs, and with blueness and congestion of the face and neck.

2   It is important first to ensure that there is a good air supply, that the mouth is not blocked with saliva or vomit.

3   Tight or restrictive clothing should be loosened.

4   If the convulsion is prolonged it can be reduced by tepid sponging of the child to bring down the temperature.

5   The child can be sponged over the body with warm water, then dried with a towel.

6   When the convulsion has stopped, if the child is not conscious, it should be placed in the coma/recovery position.

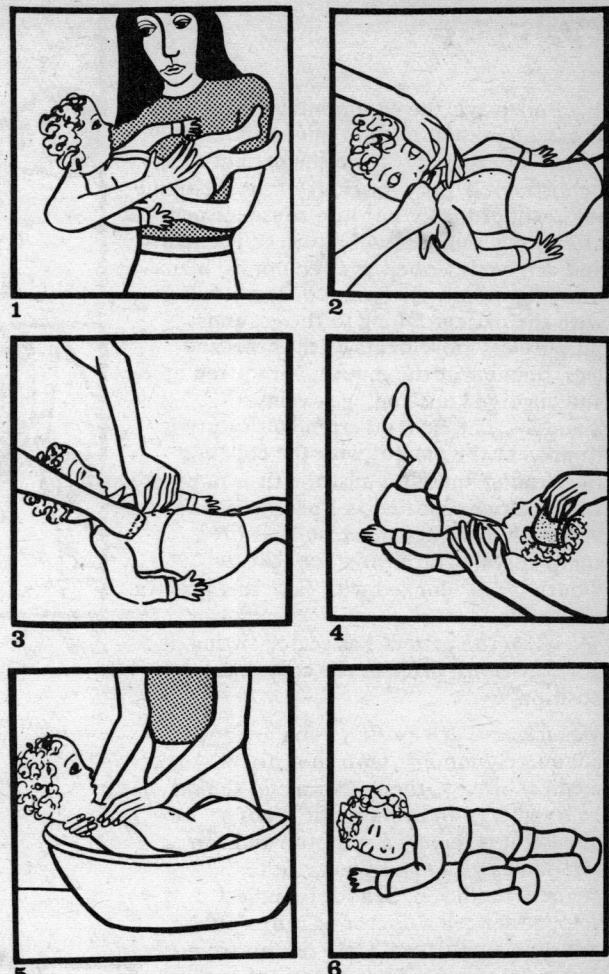

epilepsy

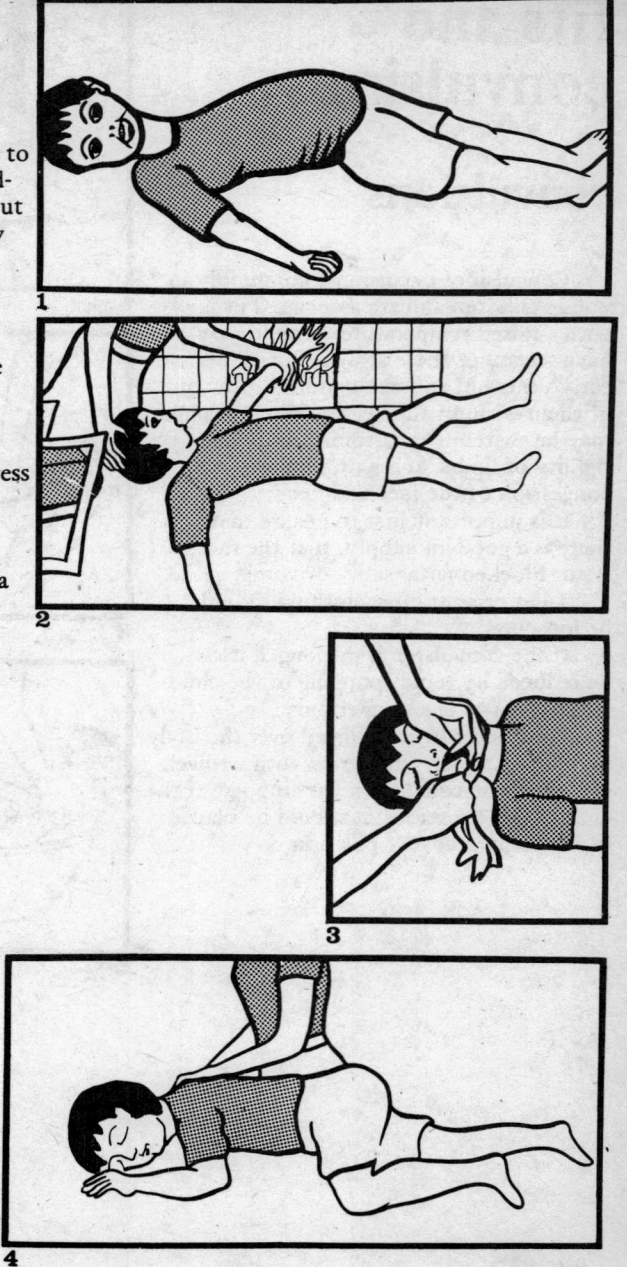

1   Epilepsy is the commonest form of fit.
It can be present both in minor and major
forms. In the minor form the patient seems to
be distracted, not conscious of his surroundings, will probably not lose consciousness but
after a few minutes will return to normality
and can be described as a temporary blank-
out. Major epilepsy (grand mal) is a full fit,
with the patient falling to the ground,
purposeless movements of the arms and
legs, foaming at the mouth, with often blue
and engorged lips and neck veins.

2 and 3   The first aid attendant's duty is
to prevent the patient with the epileptic
fit harming himself whilst the fit is in progress
and ensuring that he has a patent airway.
Protect him from danger, such as fires,
sharp edges of furniture. See that the
mouth is not blocked with false teeth, saliva
or vomit.

4   When the patient has ceased fitting, if
not conscious, place in the coma/recovery
position.

Management after a fit. If you are not
completely familiar with the patient's
medical history, then medical aid should
be sought, as an epileptic fit is not a
disease, it is merely a sympton and can
sometimes be a sign of some other
medical condition. Send for medical
help; either call a doctor or if in a public
place, an ambulance. Only refrain from
seeking medical aid when you are familiar
with both the patient and the nature of
his fits. Many patients who have epilepsy
are very embarrassed on coming round
to find themselves in hospital when they
know that they recover quickly after a
fit and feel that their hospitalisation has
been unnecessary.

   For all cases of epileptic fits that a
first aider might see, of which he has no
previous knowledge, he should carry

out the initial first aid treatment and
seek medical help, i.e. either a doctor or
an ambulance. It is not now a first aid
procedure to force a hard object between
the teeth to keep them from biting the
tongue as most people who are prone
to epileptic fits would rather have a bitten
tongue than a broken tooth.

hysterical fits

1　Hysterical fits occur usually as the
result of some emotional crisis and they
can take most forms of irrational, violent
behaviour. It is sometimes confused with
epileptic fits and varies from loss of
control with shouting and screaming to
lying on the ground, waving arms and
tearing at clothes and hair.
2　Patients with hysterical fits do not
injure themselves and the first aid attendant has to reassure them and distract
them from their exhibition by involving
them in something else, and keep them
closely under observation as, inadvertently,
they might get carried away with their
hysterical outburst and put themselves in a
situation where they could come to harm.
Occasionally a patient may have to be
slapped across the face to bring him to
his senses.

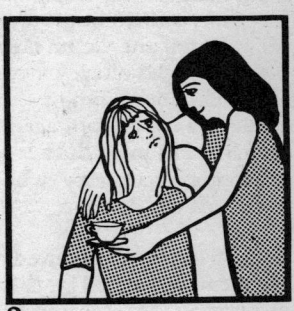

2

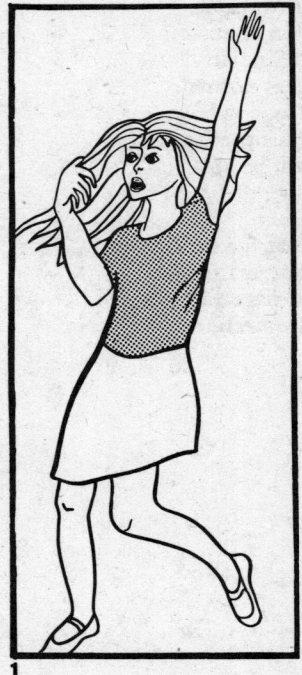

1

electrocution

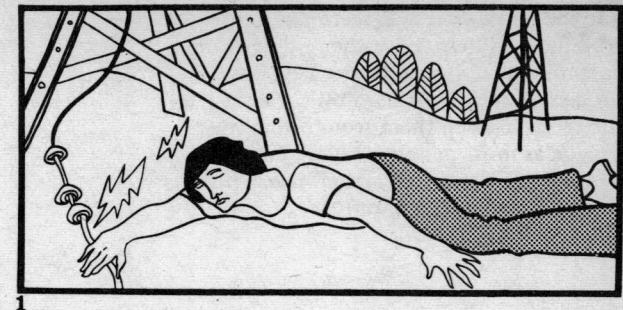

1

1   Where the electrocution is through high voltage from industrial currents, overhead electric cables, or electrified railway lines, contact may cause death immediately, the main cause of death being muscle spasm and resulting asphyxiation. It is important that the first aider should not attempt to reach the victim if the victim is still in contact with the high voltage current. Similarly, he should never climb pylons, as normal insulation is no proof against high voltage currents. His main duty is to inform the appropriate authority, who will be able to cut off the current.

If the patient has survived, treat for shock (see *Shock*, page 141), then give artificial respiration (see *Resuscitation*, page 129). Finally, treat for burns (see *Domestic Electric Burns*, page 139).

domestic
electric burns

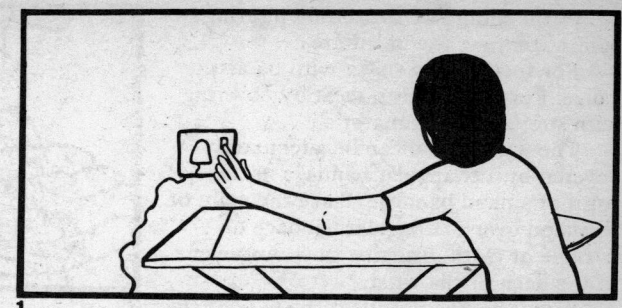

1 and 2   Electrocution from domestic electricity can be severe and can result in death. The first aider's first duty is to switch off the current that is affecting the patient by removing the plug or turning off the main switch. If it is not possible, the attendant should insulate himself and pull the patient away from his electrical contact. Rubber is the best insulation, and rubber boots or rubber-soled shoes will be enough insulation, provided they are not wet. Otherwise stand on dry insulating material, such as folded newspapers or dry wood and, using insulating material of this nature, pull the patient away from the electrical source.

Having broken the patient's contact with electricity,   treat for shock (see *Shock*, page 141), then give artificial respiration (see *Resuscitation*, page 129). Finally, treat for burns (see *Domestic Electric Burns*, page 139).

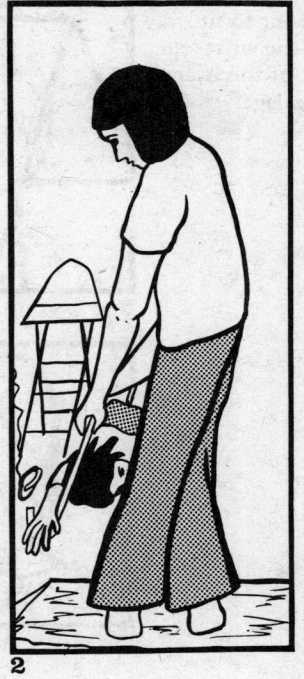

3 Burns should be treated by pouring cold water over the burnt area.

4 For small burns, cover with paraffin gauze. For larger burns, treat by covering with sterile or clean material.

5 The whole hand can be adequately covered by a triangular bandage in the form of a hand bandage. Place the palm of the hand over a triangular bandage or triangle of cloth, bringing the point over to the back of the wrist.

6 Bring the two points of the base of the triangle round to the back of the wrist, cross them and bring to the front to tie.

7 and 8 Tie on the front of the wrist and bring up the protruding point of the triangle and pin to the back of the bandage.

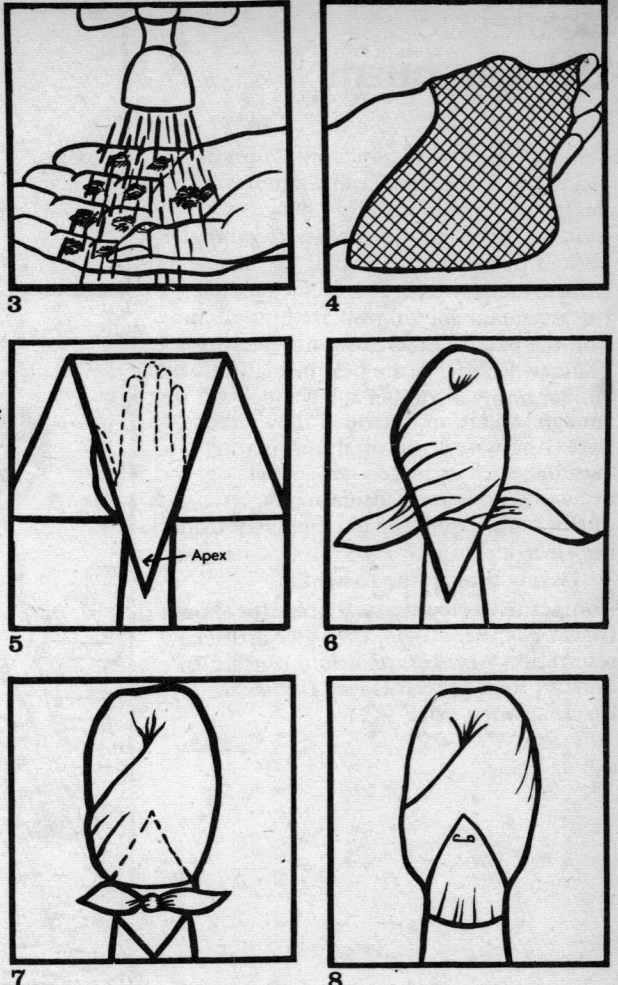

shock

Shock is a condition resulting from a collapse of many of the vital functions of the body arising from a lack of blood supply, the lack of blood supply being due to a fall in the pressure of the blood, the causes of the blood pressure falling being many. Obvious causes of lowering of the blood pressure are:
- Severe bleeding.
- Heart attacks where the heart is no longer able to pump the blood round at pressure.
- Loss of body fluids, like in severe burns, where the body is denuded of skin.
- Acute shocks to the body system, such as perforation of the stomach contents into the abdomen, or a burst appendix.
- Emotional, where news or grief can cause a complete collapse of the patient; severe pain, such as following a break of a major bone in the body or major trauma.

The symptoms of shock are common to all these conditions.

1   The patient is pale, the pulse is rapid with a poor volume, the patient is anxious, he may feel sick and may vomit, he may be giddy and have visual upsets, his breathing is usually shallow and rapid, and there may be some degree of loss of consciousness. The first aider has two duties — to treat the shock; and to ascertain the cause of the shock and, when possible, treat the cause of the situation.
2   Reassure the patient and lay him down, with his head as low as possible. Loosen tight or restrictive clothing. Keep the patient warm. Keep a close eye on the head in case of vomiting. Ascertain the cause of the shock, i.e. whether it is bleeding, perforated ulcer, or just bad news.
3   When the abdominal crises can be excluded and there is little likelihood of the patient having to have an anaesthetic, shock can be reduced by giving hot, sweet drinks by mouth.

Do not heat extremities with hot water bottles. Warm the patient generally by covering with a blanket. It is essential if there is some serious medical factor causing the shock that medical aid is sought immediately.
Emotional shock is by and large transistory, and reassurance and hot sweet drinks are usually enough to restore the situation. Do not give alcohol. Although, on occasions, people who have comfort from drink do benefit from the taking of alcohol in emotional situations, alcohol has properties that further lower the blood pressure.

4   If the shock is related to serious medical disorder, do not move the patient unless it is absolutely essential. A patient with a perforated ulcer should lie down with his head propped up, covered with a blanket, and with restrictive clothing undone at neck. He should be reassured, kept warm and observed by first aid attendant while first aid attendant is summoning medical aid.

poisoning

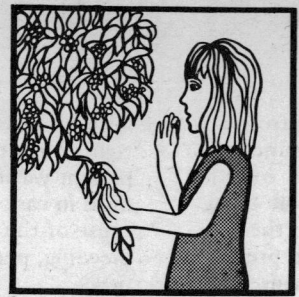

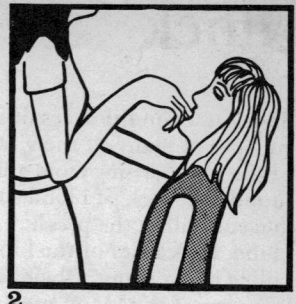

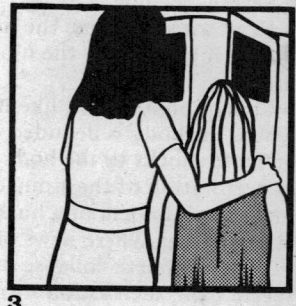

A poison is a substance which, when taken
into the body in sufficient amount, may
cause damage to health or even destroy
life. It can be liquid, solid or gaseous, and
can be taken in through the mouth by
injection, by absorption through the skin
or through the lungs through breathing.
Poisons through the mouth. The commonest
way poisons are taken into the body is
through the mouth. The commonest single
cause for admission to a medical ward of
a hospital nowadays is through self poisoning, i.e. drug overdose, either accidental
or suicidal intent.

1 and 2   Where poisoning is suspected,
first the attendant must try and get the
patient to get rid of as much poison as
possible by vomiting; secondly, the poison
must, if possible, be identified either by
collecting a specimen of vomit or looking
for possible materials that have been taken
— berries, food, or bottles of tablets — and
thirdly, the patient must be taken to a
hospital where there is a Poisons Unit.
3   ALL THE PATIENTS WHO ARE
SUSPECTED OF TAKING IN POISONS
MUST BE TAKEN TO HOSPITAL
IRRESPECTIVE OF WHETHER THEY
SHOW SYMPTOMS OR NOT as many
poisons do not start giving symptoms for
some hours after they have been taken,
and some still in fact have very toxic
effects one to two days later. Do not, as
one might see on the cinema screen, give
the patient hot coffee and walk him up
and down, hoping to get the poison out
of his system; in fact, you may be encourag-
ing the poison to be further distributed
through the body.

Poisons taken through the mouth are in two main groups — non-corrosive poisonings, and corrosive poisonings. For *non-corrosive poisons* induce the patient to vomit by putting the fingers down the back of the throat and stimulating the vomiting reflex. Do not try to make an unconscious patient vomit.

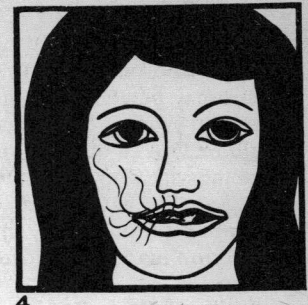

4

4   *Corrosive poisonings.* There are usually signs of burns on the lips or mouth. Unless the extent of the damage can be ascertained, the patient should not be interfered with but should be admitted to hospital as soon as possible.

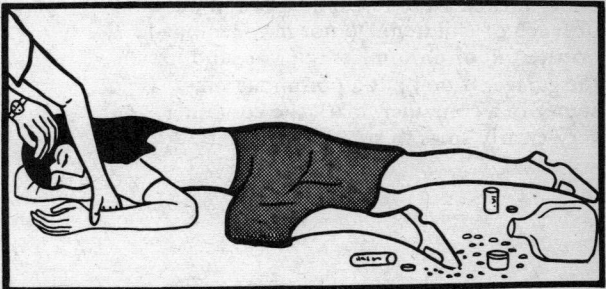

5

5   Where poisoning has caused loss of consciousness, the patient should be placed in the coma/recovery position, the pulse and respiration rates checked, and with the first aid attendant ready to commence artificial resuscitation if the condition deteriorates. The patient should be moved to hospital as soon as possible, with either specimens of vomit or other likely substances nearby that could have caused the poisoning.

Gaseous poisonings. Where gaseous poisoning is suspected, the first aid attendant must take great care that he himself is not overcome by the fumes that have poisoned the patient. The patient should first be removed from the room in which there is gas, or the room should be adequately ventilated. If the first aid attendant goes into a gas-filled room, he should open all windows and doors and then remove the patient from the gas-filled room. He should not start resuscitation procedures until he is in air that is non-toxic.

Once the patient has been removed from the presence of the toxic gas, if he does not start to recover spontaneously, resuscitation should be commenced. (See *Resuscitation*).

6 *Poisoning by injection.* Today, with the abuse and misuse of drugs, the first aider must be aware that the collapsed patient may be under the influence of drugs, and signs of drug injection marks should be looked out for, and this noted in the message sent when medical aid is requested. The patient may have syringes in his pockets, ampoules, and a pattern of injection marks and clotted veins in the arm.

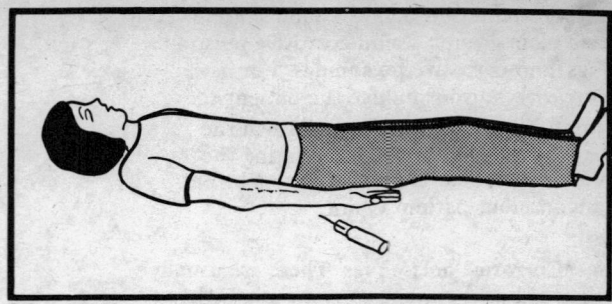

6

Avoid poisoning by keeping all poisons safely locked away in cupboards and out of reach of children. Do not have lemonade bottles full of poison left lying around the garage. If you put a poisonous substance in a container, mark the container very clearly so as to show its contents.

diabetes

The first aider should always be on the look out for sugar diabetes in patients who are behaving strangely or who are unconscious. In sugar diabetes there are two types of coma — from too much sugar, or from too much insulin, where the diabetic patient has taken insulin and not balanced it with sugar.

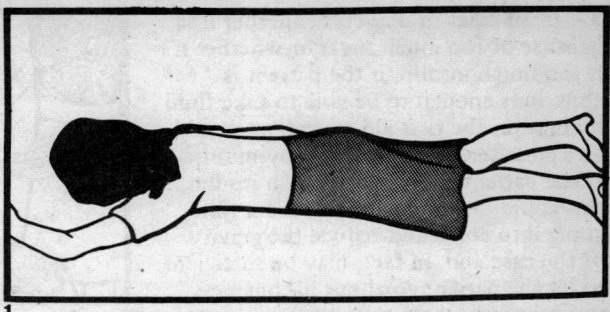

1 The first aid attendant is most likely to have to deal with the patient who has had too much insulin. The onset of coma in this situation is rapid, and the patient can often appear as if he has had too much alcohol — a little confused, unsteady on his feet, and voluble. If the patient has too much sugar in his blood, his breath will usually have the odour of pear drops, and there may be sores round the genital organs.

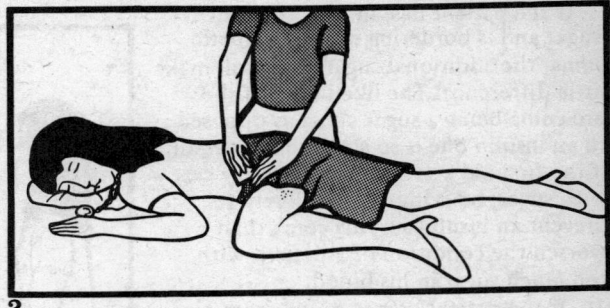

2 In all patients who are conscious or semi-conscious, and where there is no obvious cause or indication of diabetes, look for clues that the patient may be diabetic —
• A Medicalert bracelet or necklace indicating that they have diabetes;
• A diabetic card or insulin in their pocket;
• Injection marks on the upper, outer sides of the thighs or on the upper arms.

3 In all cases of diabetes, whether it is
because of too much sugar or whether it
is too much insulin, if the patient is
conscious enough to be able to take fluid
by mouth, the first aid attendant should
give glucose or sugary drinks by mouth.
If the patient has had too much insulin,
this could be sufficient to prevent him
going into coma and reduce the gravity
of the case and, in fact, may be sufficient
to let the patient go about his business
in a relatively short time.

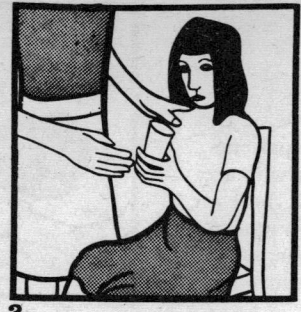

3

   If the patient has, in fact, too much
sugar and is bordering on true diabetic
coma, the additional sugar given will make
little difference. The likelihood of the
pre-coma being a sugar coma as opposed
to an insulin one is so small that, over-all,
if the first aid attendant treats every case
with sugar, he is much more likely to
prevent an insulin-surplus coma than
worsen the condition of a patient with
too much sugar in his blood.

4 If the patient comes round from his
insulin coma or insulin pre-coma, if he is
sensible and logical and is aware of the
situation he is in, there is nothing to stop
him going about his business, but unless
the first aid attendant is completely sure
that the diabetic he has been treating has
all his faculties, he should be sent immediately to hospital.

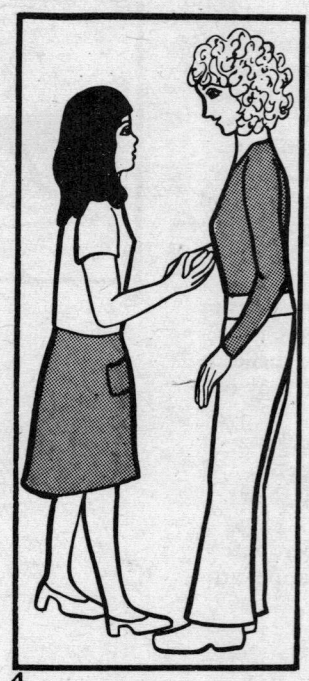

4

dog and snake bites

1   If a patient is bitten by a dog, treat the wound as a simple laceration.

2   Clean the wound well with an antiseptic solution. Controlling bleeding, if it is severe, by direct firm pressure with a pad of sterile or clean material. If the cut is large and you have some doubt as to whether it should be stitched, seek medical advice.

3   Any patient who has been bitten by a dog and has not recently had an injection for protection from the complication of tetanus, should make certain that he receives a tetanus toxoid injection within 24 hours of having been bitten. Happily rabies is not endemic in this country. If the patient is bitten in an area where rabies is endemic, then it is vitally important to seek immediate medical aid.

continued overleaf

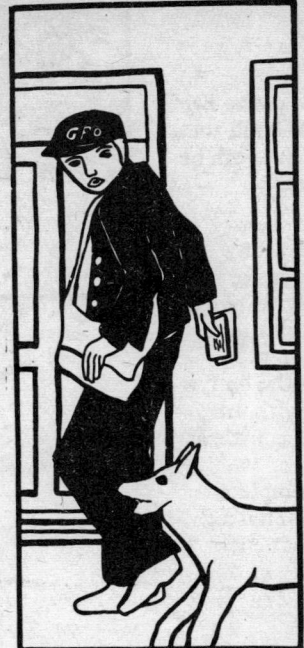

1

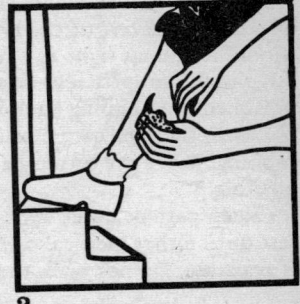

2

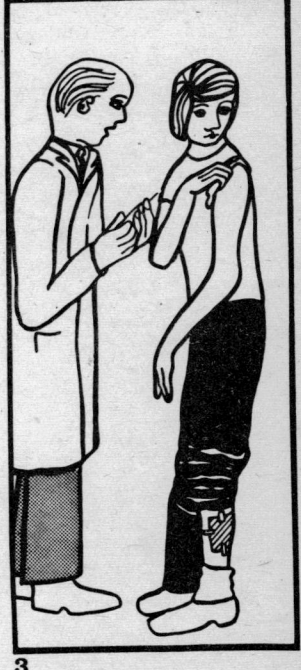

3

snake bite

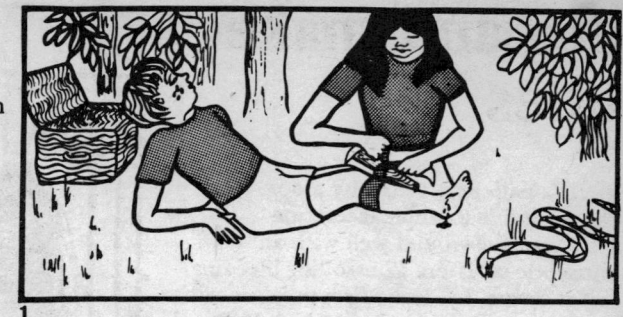

1

1   The only poisonous snake in the British Isles is the adder. When possible kill the biting snake and keep it so that it can be positively identified as an adder.

Treatment:
(a) Tie a ligature firmly around the arm or leg between where the snake has bitten and the rest of the body. Binding should not be as tight as a tourniquet, but should be sufficient to stop the poisoned blood going back in the body.
(b) Wash the area of the bite without rubbing. Move the bitten part as little as possible.
(c) Keep patient quiet with complete rest until either medical or hospital aid is available. Do not walk the patient.

drowning

The first aider's duty in a case of drowning is to get the patient from the water, get the water out of the patient, and ensure that breathing and the heart's action are normal. No time must be lost in starting resuscitation, and in drowning it is worth continuing with resuscitation for up to two hours. Do not cease resuscitation until either breathing has recommenced or a medical expert has said life is ceased.

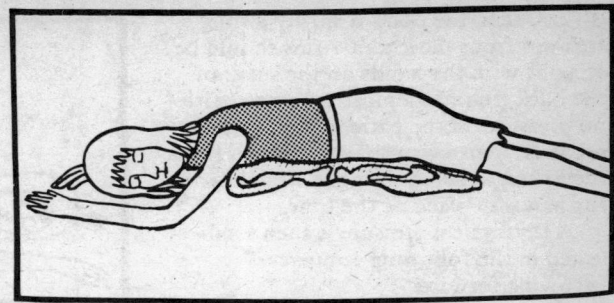

1   On removing the patient from the water, place face down, with the head on one side, and arms stretched above the head. If possible, put in a sloping position with the head at the lowest point.

For the small child or infant, hold him up by his feet for 10 or 15 seconds, then proceed as for the adult.

First raise the body by putting the hands under the stomach of the patient and lift upwards. Ensure that the airway is clear and that the mouth is not blocked by false teeth, vomit or other extraneous matter such as seaweed, weeds, etc. Loosen any restrictive clothing around the neck and waist.

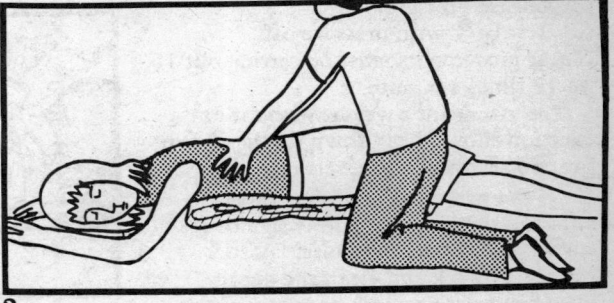

The patient should then be laid on his face with his hands folded across in front of the head, face turned on one side. Then give the patient a hard thump with the flat of the palm in the middle of the back. This can help dislodge obstructions, restart the heart or even stimulate respiration.

2   The attendant kneels on one side of the patient facing his head, the hands are placed under the small of the back of the lower ribs, the attendant sits back then so as not to put his body weight on the chest....

continued overleaf

3 . . . then the body is slowly swung forward from the knees. Arms should be straight with the hands on the small of the back, thumbs almost touching, with no pressure on the patient. Count three seconds, then swing slowly forward from the knees, keeping the arms straight and the hands in place all the time.

A rhythmical pressure is then established in the following sequence:
(a) Swing forward.
(b) Apply pressure.
(c) Release pressure.
(d) Rest back with pressure off.
These movements must be carried out 10 to 12 times a minute.

The attendant's weight without extra exertion should bear down on the patient for two seconds before relaxing.

4 If the patient is not, after three minutes, showing any visible sign of recovery and there is no pulse, lay the patient on back and clean the debris from his mouth to make a patent airway. Commence mouth-to-mouth resuscitation.

5 If the patient does not start to breathe, push up the chin and tilt the head backward.

6 Pinch the patient's nose, take a deep breath, seal your lips round the patient's mouth, blow into the lungs and watch the chest rise.

7 Stop blowing when the chest has risen, remove your mouth and watch the chest fall.

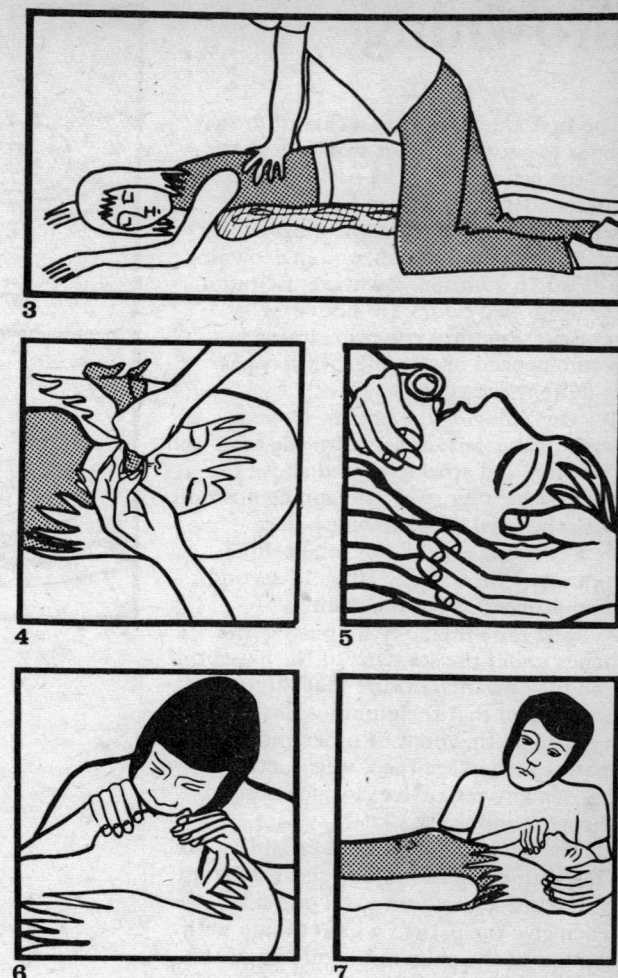

150

8 and 9   This can be continued at the normal rate of breathing until breathing is restored.

With an infant or child it is important to remember to breathe very gently or damage can be done. If the patient's heart is not beating, strike the chest smartly on the left lower part of the breast bone; if there is no response, start striking rhythmically every 10 seconds while feeling the pulse.

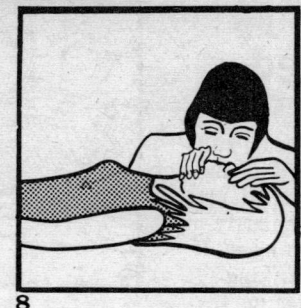 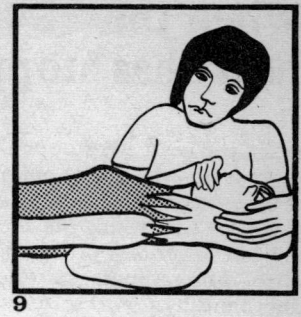

when the heart has stopped

When the heart has stopped beating and there is no evidence of pulse and the patient is blue, attempts should be made to restart the heart by striking the chest smartly on the left lower part of the breast bone. If there is no response, start by striking rhythmically for 10 seconds, feeling the pulse for evidence of re-starting of the heart. If no pulse felt, proceed to external cardiac compression. Cardiac compression should be carried out by two people, one reviving respiration and oxygenation by mouth-to-mouth resuscitation whilst the other attendant commences cardiac massage.

1   The attendant kneels at the side of the patient, facing towards the head, and puts the heel of one hand on the breast-bone with the other hand on top of it.

2   The attendant, with arms straight, should then rock forward, pressing down with firm pressure 40–60 times a minute. In children the pressure should be less and the rate higher — 60–80 times a minute.

The combination of mouth-to-mouth resuscitation and cardiac massage, if in the hands of one attendant, should be two quick lung inflations to every 14 heart compressions; if there are two first aiders, one deep lung inflation should be undertaken for every five heart compressions.

Look for recovery with an improvement of colour in the patient and pulsations in the arteries of the neck.

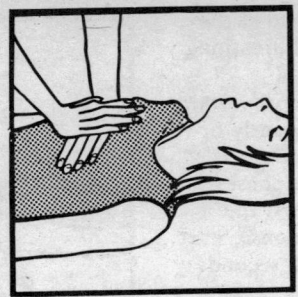
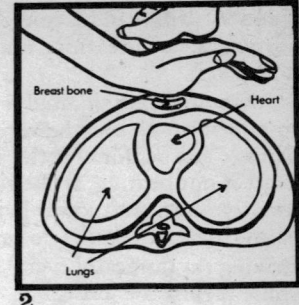

1

2

heatstroke and heat exhaustion, and the cold patient (hypothermia)

Suspect that patients who are found in a situation where there is a high temperature, with high humidity, and lack of air current and are unwell, may be suffering from heatstroke or heat exhaustion. The face is flushed and the skin hot and dry, there is a rapid pulse, noisy breathing, and the patient, if not treated, will drift into stupor and, eventually, coma. There are several contributory factors: excessive loss of fluid which is not replaced and associated loss of salt from the body in sweating, will cause upsets of the blood's chemistry, and the brain exposed to high temperature can upset the mechanism that controls the body's temperature.

The treatment is to cool the patient as quickly as possible. Remove all clothing and, if possible, wrap in a wet, cold sheet, or use a tepid sponge on the patient.

Fan him by hand or electric fan if available. If conscious, encourage him to take fluid by mouth, including some salt in the fluid.

1 If the patient is unconscious put him in the coma/recovery position, i.e. lying on one side with the underarm behind him, the upper knee bent, the lower leg very slightly bent and the upper hand lying bent in front of the face. Patients who have

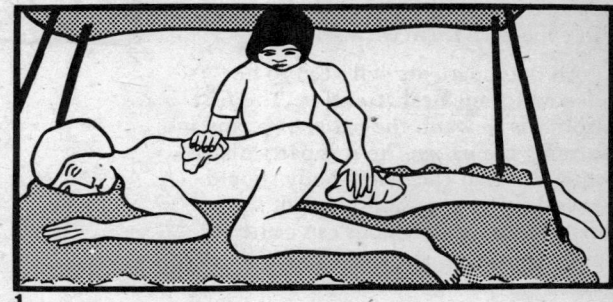

1

become unconscious with heatstroke or heat exhaustion must be referred to expert medical care, either doctor or hospital.

Prevention. Heat exhaustion and heatstroke can be prevented by-
● Wearing adequate protection to the head from the sun's rays.
● Always carrying an adequate supply of water if you are going to be exposed to excessive heat.
● Taking salt tablets by mouth as a precaution against excessive salt loss from sweating if you are going to spend some time in a hot, high humidity situation, be it desert conditions or the stoker's room in a boiler house.

2   The first aid attendant will sometimes find himself in the situation where he is confronted with a patient who has been exposed to cold, usually associated with poor nutrition, where the patient is stuporised, weak, with pulse that is difficult to feel. This occurs mainly in the elderly who have not been taking care of themselves, or in young babies who are exposed to cold conditions before they can cope with them themselves.

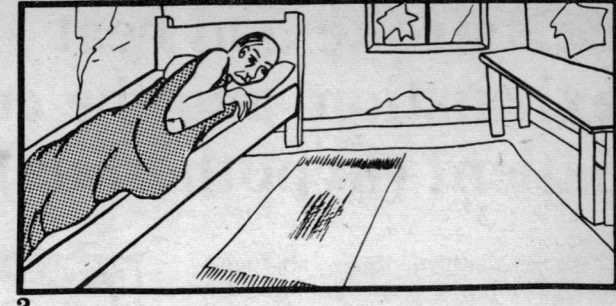

2

All these patients will need to be referred for medical attention. The first priority is to warm the patient up, and in warming the patient up it is particularly important that the whole body should be warmed as one. Applying hot water bottles to the extremities can cause complications to the already very weak patient.

Treatment:
(a) Remove any wet or sodden clothing. Cover the patient with blankets from head to foot, letting him generate his own warmth. If conscious, encourage him to drink hot, sweet drinks.
(b) Refer him for medical care and follow up.

fish hooks

1   Fish hooks — a very common injury amongst people who follow this particular sport — require special care. All fish hooks have barbs to them, and trying to withdraw the barb through its entry point will cause severe pain, damage of the surrounding tissues, and probably will not result in the removal of the fish hook.
2   Wherever possible seek medical attention where the fish hook can be removed painlessly.
3   If the patient is stoical and it is inconvenient to seek medical help, the fish hook can be removed by pushing the hook further into the finger, aiming to make the point of the hook break through the skin.
4   Then, with pliers or wire cutters, cut off the eye of the hook and its attached line.
5   Grasp the point of the hook which is protruding through the skin and pull the hook out of the finger or arm in which it is imbedded.

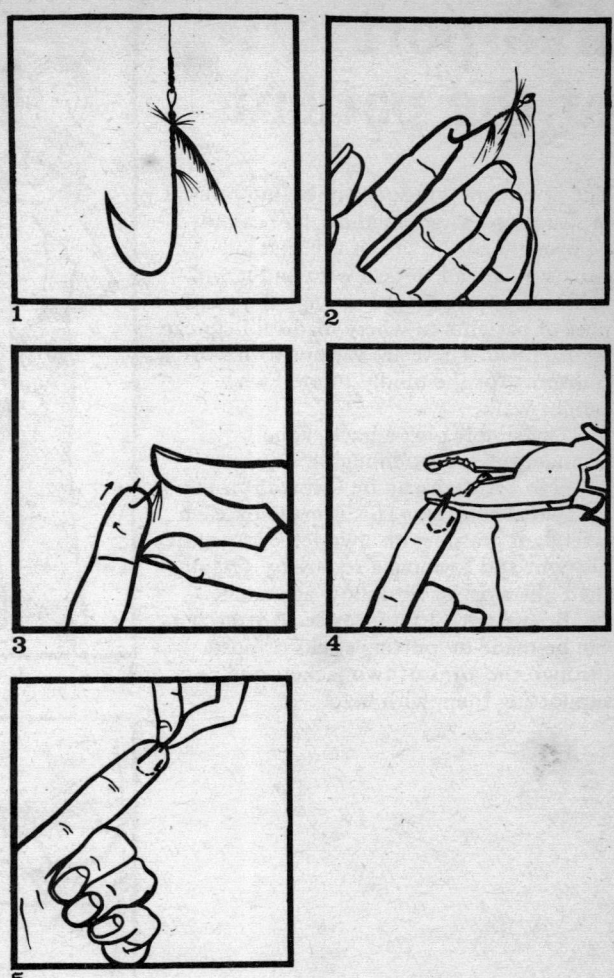

transport of the patient

The attendant will sometimes find himself in situations where medical care cannot be brought to the site of the first aid situation he had to deal with and it will be his responsibility to arrange the transport of patients to where medical help can be obtained. There are various forms of transport for the mildly injured who cannot walk:

1   The simple pick-a-back if the attendant is robust enough.

2 and 3   A chair can be formed if there are two attendants. This is made by each attendant grasping his own left wrist with his right and forming a square by grasping the right wrist of his fellow attendant.

4   Be prepared to improvise. A stretcher can be made by putting sticks or posts through the arms of two jackets and supporting them with belts.

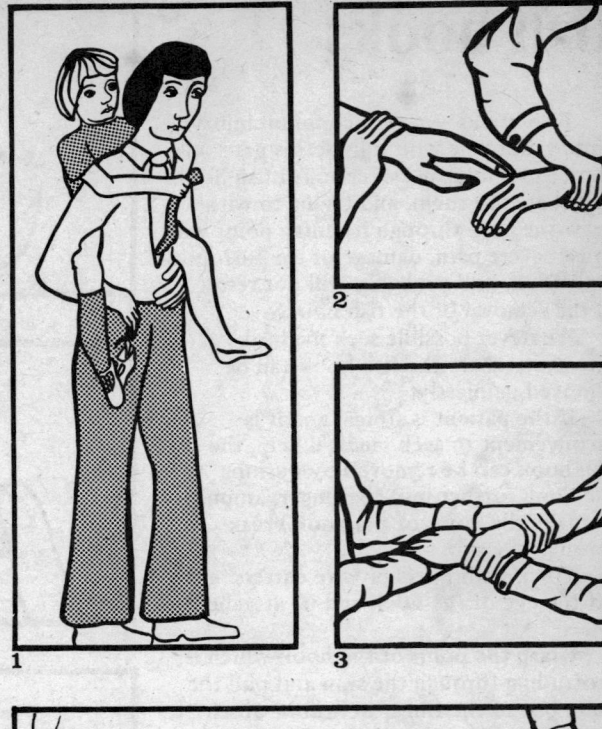

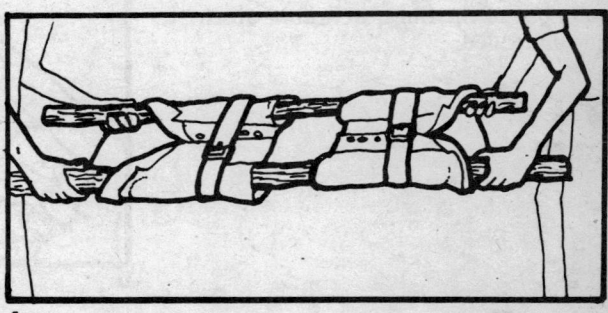

5 A plain door, if there are helpers, is often a convenient way of removing incapacitated patients until a better form of transport can be found.

6 Another sometimes neglected form of transport that can be useful in an emergency is the garden wheelbarrow. This of course will depend very much on the type of injury the patient has sustained.

Transport of patients with injured spine. Wherever possible, where it is suspected that the spine has been injured, the patient should not be moved. The body weight should be supported evenly by padding in any cavities so that there is no strain on the spine, and expert medical help should be awaited. If, however, there is no alternative to the moving of the patient, then the greatest care must be taken in the management and transporting.

7 *Transport of suspected break in the spinal column.* If it is suspected that the back is broken at any level, a stretcher must be made and brought ready next to the patient. The lifting and moving of the patient will depend very much on the number of attendants available to help in the move, and as to whether there is availability of blankets or not. Place pads of soft material between the thighs, knees and ankles of the patient.

8 Tie the ankles and feet together with figure-of-eight bandages, and tie broad bandages round the knees and thighs.

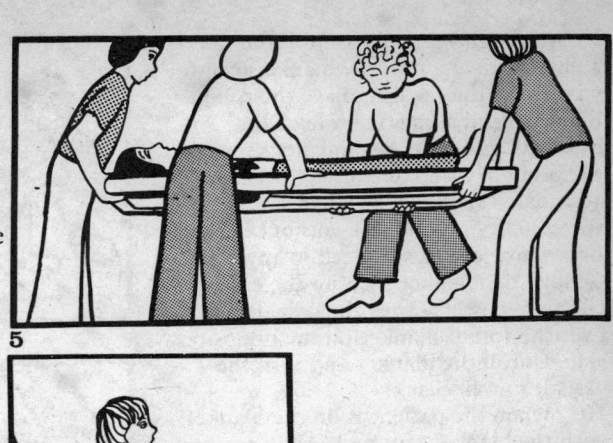

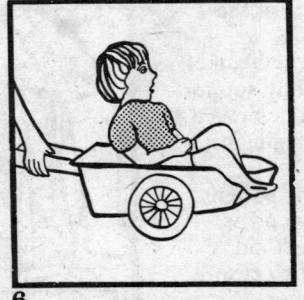

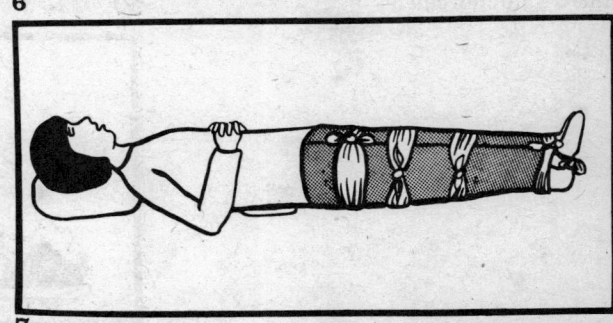

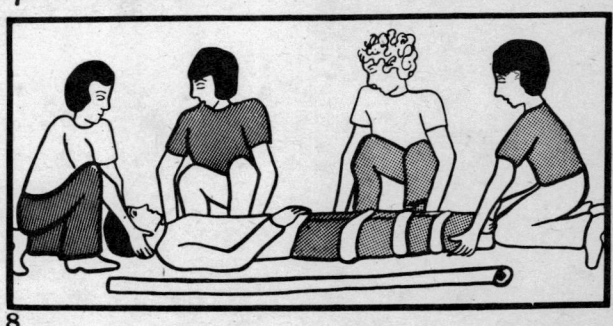

9   Where the casualty is not lying on a blanket or rug, roll the blanket lengthwise for half its width, place the roll in line with and along one side of the casualty. While two attendants keep the body in firm control, the other attendants should gently and slowly turn the casualty on one side without bending or twisting the legs or back in any way.

Move the blanket then up the casualty's back, then gently turn the casualty back over the roll of blanket on the opposite side. Unroll the blanket and turn the casualty on his back.

10   When the patient is on the blanket, with the blanket taut and firmly supporting the body, the patient can be moved on to a stretcher without changing his position.

11   Once on the stretcher the patient should be moved as smoothly and as gently as possible, with the first aid attendant being close at hand to ensure there is no movement.

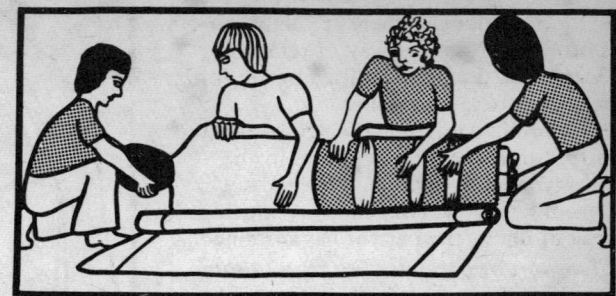

9

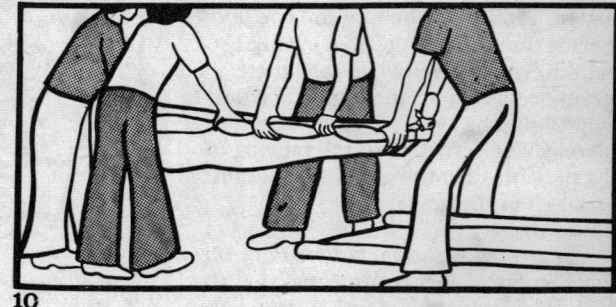

10

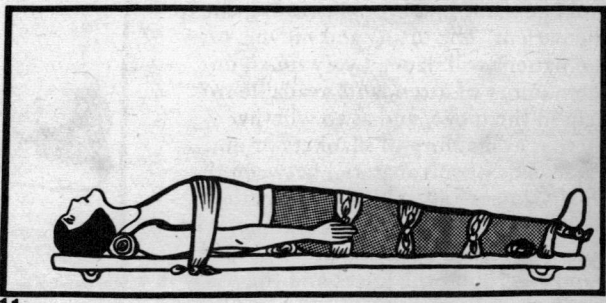

11

first aid box

All households should have at least one first aid box, and car drivers are well advised to carry a further first aid kit in their cars.

1   *The first aid cabinet.* The first aid cabinet, or box, should be clearly marked and kept in a warm, dry place which is easily accessible though out of reach of small children and known to members of the family.

It should be clearly marked with a red cross.

It is better if it is waterproof, but it need not necessarily be airtight, and should have compartments. It should shut with a firm lid or door, so that it cannot be penetrated by damp or insects, and should be childproof.

If it is to be transported, breakable containers should be adequately protected. If possible, containers should be of plastic or metal to reduce chance of breakage.

Contents of first aid box. The contents of the first aid box can vary enormously. Certain essentials are required, and, to cut down expense, many of the bandages and dressings can be made from discarded clothing material. Suggested contents:
- Tube or bottle of antiseptic lotion.
- Soluble aspirin, or Paracetamol, for relieving pain.
- 6 x 1 in. finger bandages.

- 6 x 2 in. bandages.
- 6 x 4 in. bandages.
- 2 x 3 in. crepe bandages.
- 1 x ½ in. tin zinc oxide plaster.
- 1 x 3 in. Elastoplast.
- 1 pkt. assorted sticking plaster dressings.
- 1 bottle of bicarbonate of soda.
- 1 pair scissors.
- 1 pair tweezers.
- Torch.
- Triangular bandages. (These can be made from a 3 ft. square of material, such as old sheet, by cutting diagonally across from corner to corner, giving four triangular bandages).
- Cotton wool.
- Assorted safety pins.

Useful extras for the first aid box:
- 1 tin of 10 x 10 in. paraffin gauze dressings for burns. (The author feels that these, although relatively expensive, are a very important part of a first aid box).
- Sterile pack dressings (attached to bandages and broken open for use).
- 1 plastic water bottle.
- Assorted splints, preferably inflatable ones.
- 1 indelible pencil.
- 1 roll of gauze.
- 1 bottle of old-fashioned smelling salts.